THE
Natural
Woman's
Guide TO Living
WITH THE COMPLICATIONS OF
Diabetes

M. SARA ROSENTHAL, Ph.D

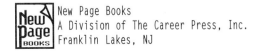
New Page Books
A Division of The Career Press, Inc.
Franklin Lakes, NJ

THE NATURAL WOMAN'S GUIDE TO LIVING WITH
THE COMPLICATIONS OF DIABETES
EDITED BY JODI BRANDON
TYPESET BY EILEEN DOW MUNSON
Cover design by Foster & Foster, Inc.
Printed in the U.S.A. by Book-mart Press

To order this title, please call toll-free 1-800-CAREER-1 (NJ and Canada: 201-848-0310) to order using VISA or MasterCard, or for further information on books from Career Press.

The Career Press, Inc., 3 Tice Road, PO Box 687,
Franklin Lakes, NJ 07417
www.careerpress.com
www.newpagebooks.com

Library of Congress Cataloging-in-Publication Data

Rosenthal, M. Sara.
    The natural woman's guide to living with the complications of diabetes / by M. Sara Rosenthal.
        p. cm.
    Includes bibliographical references and index.
    ISBN 1-56414-633-2 (pbk.)
        1. Diabetes in women—Popular works. 2. Diabetes—Complications—Prevention—Popular works. 3. Diabetes—Complications—Alternative treatment—Popular works. 4. Women—Health and hygiene—Popular works. I. Title.

RC660.4 .R685 2003
616.4'62'0082—dc21

                                                                2002034625

Important Notice

The purpose of this book is to educate. It is sold with the understanding that the author and publisher shall have neither liability nor responsibility for any injury caused or alleged to be caused directly or indirectly by the information contained in this book. Although every effort has been made to ensure its accuracy, the contents of this book should not be construed as medical advice. Each person's health needs are unique. To obtain recommendations appropriate to your particular situation, please consult a qualified healthcare provider. The herbal information in this book is provided for educational purposes only and is not meant to be used without consulting a qualified health practitioner who is trained in herbal medicine. Essential oil use is not recommended if you are pregnant or nursing. The uses of essential oils in this book are suggestions. Consult a professional for further information on dilution and usage.

Acknowledgments

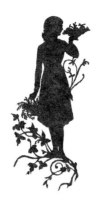

I wish to thank the following people, whose expertise and dedication helped to lay so much of the groundwork for this book (listed alphabetically): Brenda Cook, R.D., University of Alberta Hospitals; Karen Faye, L.P.N., A.F.F.A. (U.S.), Fitness Practitioner; Tasha Hamilton, Ba.Sc., R.D., Diabetes Educator-Dietitian, Tri-Hospital Diabetes Education Centre (TRIDEC); Anne Levin, B.Sc.P.T., M.C.P.A., Physiotherapist and Certified Hydrotherapist, Baycrest Centre for Geriatric Care, Coordinator, Arthritis Education and Exercise Program, and Lecturer, Physical Therapy, Faculty of Medicine, University of Toronto; Barbara McIntosh, R.N., B.Sc.N., C.D.E., Nurse Coordinator, Adult Diabetes Education Program, Grand River Hospital, Kitchener, Ontario; James McSherry, M.B., Ch.B, F.C.F.P., F.R.C.G.P., F.A.A.F.P., F.A.B.M.P., Medical Director, Victoria Family Medical Centre, Chief of Family Medicine, The London Health Sciences Centre; David Michaels, D.D.S.; Robert Panchyson, B.Sc.N., R.N., Nurse Clinician, Diabetes Educator, Hamilton Civic Hospitals, Hamilton General Division; Diana Phayre, Clinical Nurse Specialist, Diabetes Education

Centre, The Doctor's Hospital; Robert Silver, M.D., F.R.C.P.C., Endocrinologist, Division of Endocrinology and Metabolism, The Toronto Hospital.

Special thanks to Gary May, M.D., F.R.C.P., Clinical Assistant Professor of Medicine, Department of Medicine, Division of Gastroenterology, University of Calgary, and William Warren Rudd, M.D., Colon and Rectal Surgeon and Founder and Director of The Rudd Clinic for Diseases of the Colon and Rectum (Toronto), who both provided some of the groundwork for this text through their roles as medical advisors on past works. Special thanks to Mark Nesbitt, Regional Coordinator (Ontario), Canadian MedicAlert Foundation and Diabetes Patient Advocate, and Judy Nesbitt, Diabetes Patient Advocate. Endocrinologists at TRIDEC as well as several diabetes educators within the Canadian diabetes community provided their time and comments.

Gillian Arsenault, M.D., C.C.F.P., I.B.C.L.C., F.R.C.P., Simon Fraser Health Unit, served as a past advisor on two works and has never stopped advising and sending me valuable information. Irving Rootman, Ph.D., Director, Centre for Health Promotion, University of Toronto, put me in touch with several experts and always encourages my interest in primary prevention and health-promotion issues.

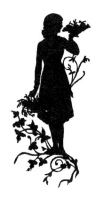

Contents

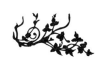

What Are Women's Diabetes Complications?

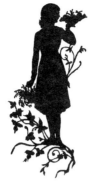

elcome to the first diabetes book devoted not only to diabetes complications in women, but one that also discusses strategies to prevent or treat these complications *naturally*, through diet, vitamin and mineral supplements, herbs, exercise, movement, and alternative systems of healing.

This is a book for women who have either:

+ Type 1 diabetes (formerly known as juvenile diabetes or insulin-dependent diabetes), which most experts believe is an autoimmune disease where the insulin-producing cells of the pancreas (the beta cells) are destroyed by the body's immune system. Ten percent of the diabetic population has Type 1 diabetes.

Or

✦ Type 2 diabetes (formerly known as adult-onset diabetes or non-insulin dependent diabetes), in which the body stops using insulin effectively or stops producing insulin. Ninety percent of the diabetic population has Type 2 diabetes. By 2004, one in four people worldwide will have Type 2 diabetes.

Of those diagnosed with Type 2 diabetes, 65 to 70 percent are women. According to some experts, about 95 percent of women with Type 2 diabetes are obese.

This is not the book to read if you have been diagnosed with gestational diabetes.

This book explains the range of complications associated with diabetes in a female body and provides you with all the information you need to *stop diabetes complications before they start*. Indeed, that is the goal of diabetes management. The most serious complications are cardiovascular, where not only heart attack and stroke are risks, but problems with your circulation can lead to amputation, mainly in the feet.

Studies on the complications of diabetes in women are sparse. Women have been traditionally underrepresented in clinical trials because of past abuses in medical research, where women sought to have their reproductive health protected. As a result, much of what we know about diabetes is based on a white, male body.

If you have previously read my book *The Type 2 Diabetic Woman*, you know that estrogen can greatly influence blood sugar control. This is the book that is your "next read," as it carefully outlines all of the complications that can occur with both types of diabetes. Diabetes can be beautifully controlled without the introduction of medication. Each chapter contains "What to Eat," "Flower Power," and "How to Move" sections that will guide you through the maze of complications that you can prevent.

If you've read my book *50 Ways Women Can Prevent Heart Disease*, you also understand how heart attacks and strokes in women are greatly increased in those who suffer from Type 2 diabetes.

More than 70 percent of all patients in the healthcare system are women; diabetes complications have a staggering impact on the healthcare system. With this book, you can begin to take your diabetes management into your own hands and make the complications of the disease manageable, too.

CHAPTER ONE

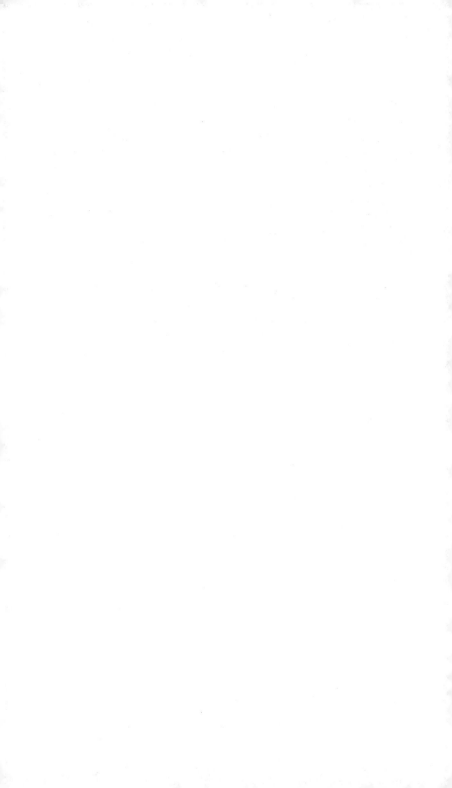

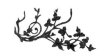

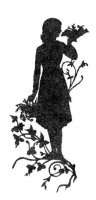

Stopping Complications Before They Start— Naturally!

If you have Type 1 diabetes (which represents 10 percent of my readers) or Type 2 diabetes (which represents 90 percent of my readers), you already know that your goal in life is to prevent the complications of either disease. You already know what diabetes means. What is absent is information about diabetes complications *for women* and *natural ways to prevent them.*

This chapter provides an overview of the various microvascular and macrovascular complications of diabetes, how they affect a woman's body, in particular, and the basic strategies you can use to avoid developing a complication from diabetes.

The Micro and the Macro

The most important thing to grasp about diabetes complications is that there are two kinds of problems that can lead to similar diseases. The first kind of problem is known as a *macrovascular complication.* The prefix *macro* means large; the word *vascular* means blood vessels (the veins and arteries that carry the blood back and forth throughout your body). Put it together, and you have large blood vessel complications. A plain-language interpretation of macrovascular complications would be "problems with your big blood vessels."

If you think of your body as a planet, a macrovascular disease would be a disease that affects the whole planet; it is body-wide, or systemic. Cardiovascular disease is a macrovascular complication that can cause heart attack, stroke, high blood pressure, and body-wide circulation problems, clinically known as peripheral vascular disease (PVD). Peripheral vascular disease refers to "fringe" blood-flow problems and is part of the heart disease story. PVD occurs when blood flow to the extremities (arms, legs, and feet) is blocked, creating cramping, pain or numbness. *In fact, pain and numbing in your arms or legs may be signs of heart disease or even an imminent heart attack.*

Macrovascular complications are caused not only by too much blood sugar, but also by preexisting health problems. People with Type 2 diabetes are far more vulnerable to macrovascular complications because they usually have contributing risk factors from way back when, such as high cholesterol and high blood pressure (both of which are discussed in Chapter 2). Obesity, smoking, and inactivity can then aggravate those problems, resulting in major cardiovascular disease and leaving the individual at risk for heart attack or stroke.

Another type of diabetes complication is known as a *microvascular complication. Micro* means tiny, as in microscopic. Microvascular complications refer to problems with the smaller blood vessels (capillaries) that connect to various body parts. A plain-language interpretation of microvascular complications would be "Houston, we've got a problem." In other words, the problem *is* serious, but it's not going to affect the whole planet, just the spacecraft in orbit. Nerve damage (neuropathy) is a microvascular complication that targets body parts such as feet, eyes, genitals, and skin. Unlike with macrovascular complications (large blood vessel complications), you're not going to have a sudden life-threatening event such as heart attack or stroke from microvascular problems. For example, eye disease (see Chapter 4), clinically known as retinopathy, is a microvascular complication. Blindness is a serious problem, but you won't die from it.

People with Type 1 diabetes are more vulnerable to microvascular complications, but a good portion of people with Type 2 diabetes suffer from them, too. Microvascular complications are known as the sugar-related complications. The small blood vessel damage is caused by high blood sugar levels over long periods of time. The Diabetes Control and Complications Trial, discussed in detail next, showed that by keeping blood sugar levels as normal as possible, *as often as possible*, through frequent self-testing, microvascular complications can be prevented.

Preventing Complications: What the Studies Show

The Diabetes Control and Complications Trial (DCCT) was a landmark study done in the 1990s that proved, without a doubt, that the road to uncomplicated diabetes is paved with frequent blood sugar monitoring. This study involved 1,441 people with Type 1 diabetes who were randomly managed according to one of two treatment philosophies: "intensive" treatment (or tight control) and "conventional" treatment (medium control). Intensive treatments involve frequently testing your blood sugar and adding a short-acting insulin that requires three to four injections daily, or one dose of longer-acting insulin. The goal of this type of management is to achieve blood sugar levels that are as normal as possible as often as possible. Conventional treatment involves controlling your diabetes to the point where you avoid feeling any symptoms of high blood sugar, such as frequent urination, thirst, or fatigue, without doing very much, if any, self-testing.

The Results

The DCCT results were unveiled in 1993 at the American Diabetes Association's annual conference. The results were pretty astounding, so much so that the trial, planned for a 10-year period, was cut short—a rare occurrence in research trials.

The people who were managed with intensive therapy were able to delay microvascular complications 36 to 76 percent of the time. Microvascular complications include nerve damage and all of the problems associated with it (see Chapter 3), eye damage (see Chapter 4), tooth decay and gum disease (see Chapter 5), kidney damage (see Chapter 6), and foot complications (see Chapter 8).

Specifically, eye disease was reduced by 76 percent, kidney disease by 56 percent, and nerve damage by 61 percent. Frequent blood sugar testing and blood sugar control also reduced high cholesterol by 35 percent, which can reduce macrovascular complications such as heart disease and stroke (see Chapter 2). *Those are very significant results.* Statistically, anything greater than 1 percent is considered "clinically significant." Wow! The overwhelming consensus among diabetes practitioners is that intensive therapy, for people with either Type 1 or Type 2 diabetes, prolongs health and greatly reduces complications.

The National Institute of Diabetes and Digestive and Kidney Diseases (NIDDK) reported similar findings when it did a similar study. NIDDK research found that with intensive therapy, eye disease was still reduced by 76 percent, kidney disease by 50 percent, nerve disease by 60 percent, and cardiovascular disease by 35 percent.

What the DCCT Means for Type 2 Diabetes

The DCCT did not look at blood sugar control and *macrovascular complications*—the cardiovascular complications (such as heart disease and stroke) for which people with Type 2 diabetes are most at risk—but it showed a significant reduction in cholesterol levels. (Natural strategies to reduce cholesterol are discussed in Chapter 2, which in turn, can reduce the risk of heart attack and stroke, which are discussed in Chapter 2.)

For several years the DCCT was controversial with Type 2 specialists. Should people with Type 2 diabetes be counseled to *intensively* control their blood sugar or not? Many specialists said that losing weight and getting diet under control are hard enough and that asking people to self-test their blood sugar three to four times per day is too much for most people with Type 2 diabetes. In other words, what's the point of avoiding microvascular complications when you're about to drop dead from a massive heart attack or stroke? Nevertheless, many specialists felt that because the DCCT showed such overwhelming reductions in complications for Type 1, until more data was out, people with Type 2 diabetes should be intensively controlling their blood sugar.

The 1998 British Study

In 1998, the results of a 20-year British study were published. Known as the United Kingdom Prospective Diabetes Study (UKPDS), it set out to determine whether blood sugar control reduces macrovascular complications in Type 2 diabetes, together with lowering blood pressure. Macrovascular complications are the cardiovascular complications, such as heart disease and stroke risk, as well as peripheral vascular disease problems, which have to do with poor blood flow to other body parts and can cause foot problems, impotence, and sexual problems for women, as well as a host of other things.

The results showed that frequent blood sugar testing can reduce the risk of blindness and kidney failure in people with Type 2 diabetes by 25 percent. In those Type 2 diabetics with high blood pressure, lowering blood pressure reduced the risk of stroke by 44 percent and of heart failure by 56 percent. And, for every one percentage point reduction in the value of the HbA$_{1c}$ test, there was a 35 percent reduction in eye, kidney, and nerve damage and an overall 25 percent reduction in deaths related to diabetes.

The bottom line is that the UKPDS shows that frequently self-testing your blood sugar can prevent long-term complications of diabetes for people with Type 2 diabetes, and, by combining that strategy with a heart-smart lifestyle, you can live well with diabetes—without complications.

Keeping Blood Sugar Stable as Often as Possible

The key to preventing all of the complications discussed in this book—naturally—is to create a meal plan with your diabetes practitioner (nutritionist, certified diabetes educator, family doctor, and so forth), stick to that meal plan, and test your blood sugar frequently. (All of this is covered later in the chapter in the "What to Eat" section.)

What Your Blood Sugar Readings Mean

In the past, three fasting blood glucose levels between 90 mg/dl (5 mmol) and 140 mg/dl (7.8 mmol) meant that you had impaired glucose tolerance (IGT). A fasting blood glucose level greater than 140 mg/dl (7.8 mol) or a random (any time of day) blood glucose level greater than 200 mg/dl (or 11.1 mmol) meant that you had diabetes.

But that's all changed. Today, anyone with a fasting blood sugar level higher than 126 mg/dl (7.0 mmol) is considered to be in the diabetic range and is officially diagnosed with diabetes. A new term, *impaired fasting glucose* (IFG), has also been introduced that refers to blood glucose levels between 110 mg/dl and 126 mg/dl (6.1 mmol and 6.9 mmol). The term IGT is now used only when describing people who have a blood glucose level between 140 mg/dl and 200 mg/dl (7. 8 and 11.1) *two hours after an oral glucose tolerance test*. Take a look at Table 1.1 for more details.

If you can't seem to keep your fasting blood sugar levels below 126 mg/dl (7.0 mmol/L), you are at risk for diabetes complications and can greatly benefit from the information in this book.

What Your Blood Sugar Readings Mean		
Fasting		
Normal	**IFG***	**Diabetes**
<110mg/dl (6.1mmol/L)	>110 mg/dl & <126 mg/dl (>6.1 mmol/L & < 7.0mmol/L)	>126mg/dl (7.0)
Two hours after an oral glucose tolerance test		
Normal	**IGT****	**Diabetes**
< 140 mg/dl (7.8 mmol/L)	>140 mg/dl & <200 mg/dl (>7.8 mmol/L - < 11.1mmol/L)	>200 mg/dl (11.1 mmol/L)
*IFG stands for impaired fasting glucose. ** IGT stands for impaired glucose tolerance, referring to test results two hours after an oral glucose tolerance test. **Note: The symbol > means "greater than"; the symbol < means "less than."**		

Table 1.1

Testing Your Own Blood Sugar

In order to plan your meals and activities properly, you have to know what your blood sugar levels are throughout the day. Glucose meters were first introduced in 1982. They allow people with diabetes to test their own blood sugar any time they want without having to rely on doctors. When your parents or grandparents struggled with diabetes in the past, there was no such thing as a glucose meter. They had to go to the doctor to get their blood sugar tested regularly. Amazingly enough, through interviews with individual diabetes patients and several doctors, my research shows that there are still people who rely on doctors to test their blood sugar. If you are still going to your doctor for a blood sugar test, purchase a glucose meter before your next doctor's visit and ask your doctor to show you how it works. There is no good reason to continue to rely on a doctor to test your blood sugar.

How Frequently Should You Test?

A healthy pancreas measures its owner's blood sugar levels once a second, or 3,600 times an hour. It produces exactly the right amount of insulin for that second. In light of this, it makes sense to test your blood sugar frequently, as confirmed by the two major studies just mentioned.

There are a host of easy-to-use home blood sugar monitors that give you more choice in diabetes self-care than ever before, so you should take advantage of them. Your doctor, pharmacist, or diabetes educator can recommend the right glucose meter for you. When you get your glucose monitor, experts suggest you compare your results to one regular laboratory test to make sure you've purchased a reliable and accurate machine.

Use the information in the boxed text that follows as a general guideline for testing times. Take it to your health care provider to help design a reasonable plan that works for you. Testing schedules are usually tailored for each individual.

When to Test Your Blood Sugar

In the days when diabetes patients went to their doctors' offices for blood sugar testing, they were usually tested first thing in the morning before eating (called a fasting blood sugar level) or immediately after eating (known as a postprandial or postmeal blood sugar level). It was believed that if either the fasting or postprandial levels were normal, the patient was stable. This is now known to be *completely false.* In fact, your blood sugar levels can bounce around all day long. Because your blood sugar is constantly changing, a blood sugar test in a doctor's office is pretty useless, because it measures what your blood sugar is only for that nanosecond. In other words, what your blood sugar is at 2:15 p.m. is not what it might be at 3:05 p.m.

It makes the most sense to test yourself before each meal, so that you know what your levels are before you eat anything, as well as about two hours after meals. Immediately after eating, blood sugar is normally high, so this is not the ideal time to test anybody. In a person without diabetes, blood sugar levels will drop about two hours after eating, in response to the natural insulin the body makes. Similarly, test yourself two hours after eating to make sure that you are able to "mimic" a normal blood sugar pattern, too. Ideally, this translates into at least four blood tests daily:

1. When you wake up

2. After breakfast/before lunch (two hours after breakfast)

3. After lunch/before dinner (two hours after lunch)

4. After dinner/or at bedtime (two hours after dinner)

When to Test Your Blood Sugar (cont.)

The most revealing information about your blood sugar control is in the answers to the following questions:

1. What is your blood sugar level as soon as you wake up? (In people with Type 2 diabetes, it is often at its highest point in the morning.)

2. What is your blood sugar level two hours *after* a meal? (It should be much lower two hours after eating than one hour after eating.)

3. What is your blood sugar level when you feel ill? (You need to avoid dipping too low or high because your routine is changing.)

Variations on the theme:

✧ Test yourself four times a day (times indicated previously in this box) two to three times a week, and then test yourself two times a day (before breakfast and before bedtime) for the remainder of the week.

✧ Test yourself twice a day three to four days a week in a rotating pattern (before breakfast and dinner one day, before lunch and bedtime the next).

✧ Test yourself once a day every day, but rotate your pattern (day 1 before breakfast, day 2 after dinner, day 3 before bedtime, and so on).

✧ Test yourself four times a day (times indicated previously in this box) two days a month.

A Brief History of Blood Sugar Tests

At one time, the only way you could test your blood sugar level yourself was to test your urine for sugar. If the result showed that sugar was in your urine, you had already reached your renal threshold (kidney limit). Renal thresholds vary between 110 mg/dl and 200 mg/dl (6.1 and 11 mmol/L), but the limitations of urine testing were that it could only test for *really* high blood sugar levels and the results were delayed, meaning that you could be getting readings on urine that had been in the bladder for hours versus "fresh" urine (urine that has been in the bladder for less than an hour). Urine testing is also useless for checking low blood sugar. Far more accurate home blood sugar testing became available with the development of glucose meters in 1982, but the first meters were very expensive (about $600). Thankfully, meters today are quite affordable.

The first models measured glucose levels in whole blood, whereas laboratories were still measuring glucose levels in blood plasma. The difference is technical and not important to you personally. What you need to know, however, is that the readings varried. This meant that doctors needed to add about 12 percent to the glucose meter's recordings in order to get an accurate picture. This standard has changed. Today, all glucose meters measure glucose levels in plasma. If you're using an older glucose meter, don't panic when your next glucose meter suddenly gives you readings that are 12 percent higher than your last meter. It doesn't mean that you are losing control of your diabetes; rather, your meter is measuring glucose levels in your plasma instead of whole blood. Some diabetes literature recommends that you ask the pharmacist if the meter is a whole-blood test or a plasma test, but most diabetes educators will tell you that this question is pretty redundant these days as all glucose meters are now plasma tests.

Choosing and Using Your Glucose Meter

As in the computer industry, glucose meter manufacturers tend to come out with technological upgrades every year. In fact, newer models allow you to download the time, date, and blood sugar values for as many as 250 tests right onto your personal computer or personal organizer device. The information can help you gauge whether your diet and exercise routine is working or whether you need to adjust your medications or insulin. If you've never purchased a glucose meter, keep in mind that the lowest-tech glucose meters all provide the following:

+ A battery-powered, pocket-sized device.
+ An LED or LCD screen (that is, a calculator-like screen).
+ Accurate results in seconds.
+ At least a one-year warranty.
+ The opportunity to upgrade.
+ A 1-800 customer service hotline.
+ Mailings and giveaways every so often.
+ A few free lancets with your purchase. You may have to separately purchase a lancing device, a dispenser for your lancets; eventually, you'll run out of lancets and have to buy those, too.

The directions for using a glucose meter vary according to manufacturer. Be sure to read the directions carefully and ask your pharmacist for guidance if there's something you don't understand. It's a good idea to record your results in a logbook.

Factors That Can Taint Your Results

Keep in mind that the following outside factors may interfere with your meter's performance.

Other medications you're taking. Studies show that some meters can be inaccurate if you're taking acetaminophen, salicylate, ascorbic acid, dopamine, or levodopa. As a rule, if you're taking any medications, check with your doctor, pharmacist, and glucose meter manufacturer (call their 1-800 number) about whether your medications can affect the meter's accuracy.

Humidity. The worst place to keep your meter and strips is in the bathroom where humidity can ruin your strips, unless they're individually wrapped in foil. Keep your strips in a sealed container away from extreme temperatures. Don't store your meter and strips, for example, in a hot glove compartment; don't keep them in the freezer either.

Bright light. Ever tried to use a calculator or portable computer in bright sunlight? It's not possible, because the light interferes with the screen. Some meters are photometric, which means they are affected by bright light. If you plan to test in sunlight, get a biosenser meter that is unaffected by bright light (several exist).

Touching the test strip. Many glucose meters come with test strips that cannot be touched with your fingers or a second drop of blood. If you're all thumbs, purchase a meter that is unaffected by touch and/or allows a second drop of blood.

Wet hands. Before you test, thoroughly dry your hands. Water can dilute your blood sample.

Motion. It's always best to test yourself when you're standing still. Testing on planes, trains, automobiles, buses, and subways may affect your results, depending on the brand of glucose meter.

Dirt, lint, and blood. Particles of dirt, lint, and old blood can sometimes affect the accuracy of a meter, depending on the brand. Make sure you clean the meter regularly (follow the manufacturer's cleaning directions) to remove buildup. If your meter requires battery changes, make sure you change them! There are meters on the market that do not require cleaning and are unaffected by dirt, but they may cost a little more.

Glycosylated Hemoglobin

The most detailed blood sugar test cannot be done at home yet. This is a blood test that checks for glycosylated hemoglobin (glucose attached to the protein in your red blood cells), known as *glycohemoglobin* or HbA_{1c} levels. This test can tell you how well your blood sugar has been controlled over a period of two to three months by showing what percentage of it is too high. All diabetes associations recommended that you get an HbA_{1c} test every three months.

Preventing High Blood Sugar

Common reasons for a change in blood sugar levels revolve around the following:

+ Overeating or eating more than usual.

+ A change in exercise routine.

+ Missing a medication dose or an insulin shot (if you're taking insulin).

+ An out-of-the-ordinary event (illness, stress, upset, excitement).

+ A sudden mood change (extreme fright, anger, or sadness).

+ Pregnancy.

In response to unusual strains or stress, your body taps into its stored glucose supplies for extra energy. This will raise your blood sugar level, as more glucose than usual is released into your system. Whether you're fighting off a flu or fighting with your mother, digesting all that food you ate at that all-you-can-eat buffet or running away from a black bear, your body will try to give you the extra boost of energy you need to get through your immediate stress.

Blood sugar levels naturally rise when you're ill. In the event of a cold, fever, flu, or injury, you'll need to adjust your routine to accommodate high blood sugar levels, especially if vomiting or diarrhea is occurring. In some cases, you may need to go on insulin temporarily.

Preventing Low Blood Sugar

Preventing low blood sugar is equally important. Hypoglycemia can sometimes come on suddenly, particularly overnight, because blood sugar can drop while you sleep. Planning your meals around your activity should prevent episodes of low blood sugar.

Any blood sugar reading below 70 mg/dl (3.8 mmol/L) is considered too low. A hypoglycemic episode is characterized by two stages: the warning stage and what I call the *actual* hypoglycemic episode. The warning stage occurs when your blood sugar levels *begin* to drop and can occur as early as a blood sugar reading of 108 mg/dl (6 mmol/L) in people with typically higher than normal blood sugar levels. When your blood sugar drops below 55 mg/dl (or 3 mmol/L) you are *officially* hypoglycemic.

If you can begin to recognize the warning signs of hypoglycemia, you may be able to stabilize your blood sugar before you lose consciousness. Most people will notice feeling hungry and headachy, then sweaty, nervous, and dizzy. Those who live with or spend a lot of time with you should learn to notice sudden mood changes (usually extreme irritability, "drunklike aggression," and confusion) as a warning that you are "low." Whether you notice your own mood changes or not, you, too, will feel suddenly unwell. By simply asking yourself, "Why is this happening?" you should be able to remember that it's a warning that your blood sugar is low and reach for your snack pack (see p. 49 later in the chapter). The irritability can simulate the rantings of someone who is drunk; the weakness and shakiness can lead to the lack of coordination seen in someone who is drunk. For this reason, it's crucial that you carry a card or wear a bracelet that identifies that you have diabetes.

Hypoglycemia is serious: If left untreated, hypoglycemia can also result in coma, brain damage, and death. Hypoglycemia is considered the official cause of death in about 5 percent of the Type 1 diabetic population, and in the past, hypoglycemia was a more common problem among people with Type 1 diabetes. But because 40 to 50 percent of all people with Type 2 diabetes will eventually graduate to insulin therapy, the incidence of hypoglycemia has increased by 300 percent in this group. Moreover, hypoglycemia is a common side effect of oral hypoglycemic pills, the medication the majority of people with Type 2 take when they are first diagnosed.

An episode of hypoglycemia can be triggered by:

✦ Delaying or missing a meal or snack (see "What to Eat").

✦ Drinking alcohol (see Chapter 2).

✦ Exercising too long or strong (without compensating with extra food; see Chapter 2).

Low blood sugar can also be the result of too high an insulin dose, which is what is meant by the term *insulin shock* (or insulin reaction). This is a misleading term, however, because it implies that only people who take insulin can become hypoglycemic.

How to Handle an Episode of Low Blood Sugar

No one with diabetes is immune to hypoglycemia; it can occur in someone with long-standing diabetes just as much as in someone newly diagnosed. The important thing is to be alert to the warning signs. Not everyone experiences the same warning symptoms, but here are some signs to watch for:

✦ Pounding, racing heart.

✦ Breathing fast.

✦ Skin turning white.

✦ Sweating (cold sweat in big drops).

- Trembling, tremors, or shaking.
- Goose bumps or pale, cool skin.
- Extreme hunger pangs.
- Light-headedness (feeling dizzy or that the room is spinning).
- Nervousness, extreme irritability, or a sudden mood change.
- Confusion.
- Feeling weak or faint.
- Headache.
- Vision changes (seeing double or blurry vision).

Some people will experience no symptoms at all. If you've had a hypoglycemic episode without any warning symptoms, it's important for you to eat regularly and to test your blood sugar. If you're experiencing frequent hypoglycemic episodes, diabetes educators recommend that by keeping your sugar above normal, you can prevent low blood sugar. In some cases of long-standing diabetes and repeated hypoglycemic episodes, experts note that the warning symptoms may not always occur. Experts in the diabetes community believe that in some people, the body eventually loses its ability to detect hypoglycemia and send adrenaline. Furthermore, if you've switched from an animal to human insulin, warning symptoms may not be as pronounced.

WHAT TO EAT

Managing diabetes and blood sugar levels and preventing complications revolve solely around what to eat in terms of your meal plan. In chapters specific to certain complications, I will tailor this information to the specific complication you want to prevent (or refer you back to this section). There is a lot of anecdotal evidence surrounding the benefits of certain nutritional supplements such as chromium, discussed later. Fiber is also essential in keeping blood sugar levels stable (see page 43).

Meal plans are recommended by registered dietitians and are tailored to your individual goals and medication regimen. The goal is to keep the supply of glucose consistent by spacing out your meals, snacks, and activity levels accordingly. If you have Type 2 diabetes and lose weight, this will allow your body to use insulin more effectively, but not all people with Type 2 diabetes need to lose weight. If you're on insulin, meals will have to be timed to match the peak of your insulin. A dietitian can be helpful by prescribing an individualized meal plan that addresses your specific needs (weight control, shift work, travel, and so forth).

A good meal plan will ensure that you are getting enough nutrients to meet your energy needs and that your food is spread out over the course of the day. For example, if your meal plan allots for three meals with one to two snacks; meals should be spaced four to six hours apart so your body isn't overwhelmed. If you are obese, snacks will likely be discouraged because snacks can cause you to oversecrete insulin and increase your appetite. A meal plan should also help you to eat consistently rather than binging one day and starving the next.

A good meal plan will also ensure that you're getting the vitamins and minerals you need without taking supplements, such as iron, calcium, folic acid, vitamins A, B_1, B_2, B_3, C, D, and E. (See Appendix A for food sources of these vitamins.)

Golden Rules of Diabetes Meal Plans

+ Eat three meals a day at fairly regular times (spaced four to six hours apart).

+ Try to eat a variety of foods each day from all food groups.

✦ Ask your dietitian to help you plan your snacks.

✦ Learn how to gauge serving sizes, volume of bowls and glasses, and so on.

✦ Ask your dietitian or diabetes educator about how to adjust your diet if you're traveling. (This will depend on whether you're on medication, where you're going, what foods will be available, and so on.)

✦ Draw up a sick-days plan with your dietitian. (This will depend on what your regular meal plan includes.)

✦ Ask about any meal supplements, such as breakfast bars, sports bars, or meal replacement drinks.

✦ Choose lower fat foods more often.

Understanding Carbs

Carbohydrates are like people; they can be simple or complex. Simple carbohydrates are found in any food that has natural sugar (honey, fruits, juices, vegetables, milk) and anything that contains table sugar or sucrose.

Complex carbohydrates are more sophisticated foods that are made up of larger molecules, such as grain foods, starches, and foods high in fiber. (The fiber foods, such as cereals, oatmeal, or legumes, and the important between soluble and insoluble, are topics discussed later in this book.)

The Glycemic Index

The glycemic index (GI) shows the rise in blood sugar from various carbohydrates. Therefore, planning your diet using the GI can help you control your blood sugar by using more foods with a low GI and fewer foods with a high GI. Encouraging people with IGT or Type 2 diabetes to use the GI is now recommended by diabetes organizations worldwide.

The Glycemic Index at a Glance

Sugars

Glucose = 100
Honey = 87
Table sugar = 59
Fructose = 20

Snacks

Mars bar = 68
Potato chips = 51
Sponge cake = 46
Fish sticks = 38
Tomato soup = 38
Sausages = 28
Peanuts = 13

Cereals

Cornflakes = 80
Shredded Wheat = 67
Muesli = 66
All Bran = 51
Oatmeal = 49

Breads

Whole wheat = 72
White = 69
Buckwheat = 51

Fruits

Raisins = 64
Banana = 62
Orange juice = 46
Orange = 40
Apple = 39

Dairy Products

Ice cream = 36
Yogurt = 36
Milk = 34
Skim milk = 32

Root Vegetables

Parsnips = 97
Carrots = 92
Instant mashed potatoes = 80
New boiled potato = 70
Beets = 64
Yam = 51
Sweet potato = 48

Pasta and Rice

White rice = 72
Brown rice = 66
Spaghetti (white) = 50
Spaghetti (whole wheat) = 42

Legumes

Frozen peas = 51
Baked beans = 40
Chickpeas = 36
Lima beans = 36
Butter beans = 36
Black-eyed peas = 33
Green beans = 31
Kidney beans = 29
Lentils = 29
Dried soybeans = 15

Source: Adapted from David Drum and Terry Zierenberg, R.N., CDE, *The Type 2 Diabetes Sourcebook.* (Los Angeles: Lowell House, 1998), p. 130. Used with permission.

> ## The Glycemic Index at a Glance
>
> This glycemic index, developed at the University of Toronto, measures the rate at which various foods convert to glucose, which is assigned a value of 100. Higher numbers indicate a more rapid absorption of glucose. This is not an exhaustive list and should be used as a *sample* only. This is not an index of food energy values or calories; some low GI foods are high in fat, and some high GI foods are low in fat. Keep in mind, too, that these values differ depending on what else you're eating with that food and how the food is prepared.

Table 1.2

The Exchange System

The first thing you need to learn before you shop for food is the exchange system, developed by the American Diabetes Association, which will tells you how various foods can be incorporated into your meal plan. (This is different than the Food Choice Value System symbols used by the Canadian Diabetes Association, in case you're shopping in Canada.) There are seven exchange list categories:

I. Starches List.
>   Includes cereals, grains, pasta, breads, crackers, snacks, and starchy vegetables, such as legumes (peas and beans), potatoes, corn, and squash.

II. Meat and Meat Substitutes List.
>   Includes poultry, fish, shellfish, game, beef, pork, lamb, cheese, tofu, tempeh, low-fat cheeses, egg whites, and soy milk.

III. Fruit List.
>   Includes fresh fruit, frozen fruit, canned fruit, dried fruit, and juice. (*Remember: Fruit is any produce that grows on trees/vines/plants, such as tomatoes.*)

IV. Dairy List.
Includes most milk products.

V. Vegetable List.
Includes most vegetables from A (for artichoke) to Z (for zucchini), but does *not* include starchy vegetables. (See Starches List.)

VI. Fats List.
Includes monounsaturated fats, polyunsaturated fats, and saturated fats, based on the main type of fat any food contains.

VII. Other Carbohydrates.
Includes cakes, pies, puddings, granola bars, gelatin, and so forth. This list includes any food that contains more fats and sugars than vitamins and minerals.

Your dietitian or diabetes educator will work with you to create an individual meal plan built around the just-described exchange lists. One person, for example, may eat for breakfast: two items from List I, three items from List II, and two items from List VI; another person may require a completely different plan. I cannot tell you, in this book, how many items from the above lists you can have; I can only explain *how* the foods are categorized.

Your dietitian or diabetes educator should also teach you how to incorporate *carbohydrate counting* ("carb counting") into meal planning, which can be done by learning to read labels properly, setting goals for a certain number of carbohydrates per day, and keeping accurate records of your blood sugar levels.

The best advice regarding exchange lists is to purchase The American Diabetes Association's *Exchange Lists for Meal Planning* (the exchange list bible). It can be ordered directly from the American Diabetes Association by calling (800) 232-6733.

How Your Food Breaks Down

Use this table as a guideline to determine how fast your food breaks down, so you can plan for your meals better.

Complex Carbohydrates (digest more slowly)	**Defined by ADA**
fruits	Fruit List
vegetables (corn, potatoes, etc.)	Vegetables List or Starches List
grains (breads, pastas, and cereals)	Starches List
legumes (dried beans, peas, and lentils)	Starches List

Simple Carbohydrates (digest quickly)	**Defined by ADA**
fruits/fruit juices	Fruit List
sugars (sucrose, fructose, etc.)	Fruit/Other Carbohydrates/ Starches Lists
honey	Fruit/Other Carbohydrates/ Starches Lists
corn syrup	Fruit/Other Carbohydrates/ Starches Lists
sorghum	Fruit/Other Carbohydrates/ Starches Lists
date sugar	Fruit/Other Carbohydrates/ Starches Lists
molasses	Fruit/Other Carbohydrates/ Starches Lists
lactose	Dairy List

How Your Food Breaks Down (cont.)

Proteins (digest slowly)	**Defined by ADA**
lean meats	Meat and Meat Substitutes List
fatty meats	Meat and Meat Sub/Fats lists
poultry	Meat and Meat Substitutes List
fish	Meat and Meat Substitutes List
eggs	Meat and Meat Substitutes List
low-fat cheese	Meat and Meat Substitutes List
high-fat cheese	Dairy List or Fats List
legumes	Starches List
grains	Starches List

Fats (digest slowly)	**Defined by ADA**
high-fat dairy products (butter or cream)	Dairy List or Fats List
oils (canola/corn/olive/ safflower/sunflower)	Fats List
lard	Fats List
avocados	Fats List or Vegetable List
olives	Fats List or Vegetable List
nuts	Fats List or Vegetable List
fatty meats	Fats/ Meat and Meat Substitutes Lists

Fiber (doesn't digest; goes through you)	**Defined by ADA**
whole-grain breads	Starches List
cereals (such as oatmeal)	Starches List
all fruits	Fruit List
legumes (beans, lentils)	Starches List
leafy greens	Vegetable List
cruciferous vegetables	Vegetable List

Table 1.3

Understanding Sugar

Sugars are found naturally in many foods you eat. The simplest form of sugar is glucose, which is what "blood sugar," also called "blood glucose," is: your basic body fuel. You can buy pure glucose at any drugstore in the form of dextrose tablets. Dextrose is just "edible glucose." For example, when you see people having "sugar water" fed to them intravenously, dextrose is the sugar in that water. When you see dextrose on a candy-bar label, it means that the candy-bar manufacturer used edible glucose in the recipe.

Glucose is the baseline ingredient of all naturally occurring sugars, which include:

+ Sucrose: table or white sugar, naturally found in sugar cane and sugar beets.

+ Fructose: the natural sugar in fruits and vegetables.

+ Lactose: the natural sugar in all milk products.

+ Maltose: the natural sugar in grains (flours and cereals).

When you ingest a natural sugar of any kind, you're actually ingesting one part glucose and one or two parts of *another* naturally occurring sugar. For example, sucrose is biochemically constructed from one part glucose and one part fructose. So from glucose it came, and unto glucose it shall return—once it hits your digestive system. The same is true for all naturally occurring sugars, with the exception of lactose. As it happens, lactose breaks down into glucose and an "odd duck" simple sugar, galactose (which I used to think was something in our solar system, until I became a health writer). Just think of lactose as the "milky way" and you'll probably remember.

Simple sugars can get pretty complicated when you discuss their molecular structures. For example, simple sugars can be classified as monosaccharides (a.k.a. single sugars) or dissaccharides (a.k.a. double sugars). But unless you're writing a chemistry exam on sugars, you don't need to know this confusing stuff: You just need to know that all naturally occurring sugars wind up as glucose once you eat them; glucose is carried to your cells through the bloodstream and is used as body fuel or energy.

How long does it take for one of these sugars to return to glucose? Well, it greatly depends on the amount of fiber in your food, how much protein you've eaten, and how much fat accompanies the sugar in your meal. If you have enough energy or fuel, once that sugar becomes glucose, it can be stored as fat. And that's how—and why—sugar can make you fat.

Factory-Added Sugars

What you have to watch out for is *added sugar,* sugars that manufacturers add to foods during processing or packaging. Foods containing fruit juice concentrates, invert sugar, regular corn syrup, honey, molasses, hydrolyzed lactose syrup, or high-fructose corn syrup (made out of highly concentrated fructose through the hydrolysis of starch) all have added sugars. Many people don't realize, however, that pure, *unsweetened* fruit juice is still a potent source of sugar, even when it contains no added sugar. Extra lactose (naturally occurring sugar in milk products), dextrose (edible glucose), and maltose (naturally occurring sugar in grains) are also contained in many of your foods. In other words, the products may have naturally occurring sugars anyway, and then *more* sugar is thrown in to enhance consistency, taste, and so on. The best way to know how much sugar is in a product is to look at the nutritional label for carbohydrates.

Understanding Sweeteners

We gravitate toward sweet flavors because we start out with the slightly sweet taste of breast milk. A product can be sweet without containing a drop of sugar, thanks to the invention of artificial sugars and sweeteners. Artificial sweeteners will not affect your blood sugar levels because they do not contain sugar; they may contain a very few calories, however. It depends on whether that sweetener is classified as nutritive or non-nutritive.

Nutritive sweeteners have calories or contain natural sugar. White or brown table sugar, molasses, honey, and syrup are all considered nutritive sweeteners. *Sugar alcohols* are also nutritive sweeteners because they are made from fruits or produced commercially from dextrose. Sorbitol, mannitol, xylitol, and maltitol are all sugar alcohols. Sugar alcohols contain only four calories per gram, as ordinary sugar does, and will affect your blood sugar levels the way ordinary sugar does. How much sugar alcohols affect your blood sugar levels all depends on how much is consumed and the degree of absorption from your digestive tract.

Non-nutritive sweeteners are sugar substitutes or artificial sweeteners; they do not have any calories and will not affect your blood sugar levels. Examples of non-nutritive sweeteners are saccharin, cyclamate, aspartame, sucralose, and acesulflame potassium.

The oldest non-nutritive sweetener is saccharin, which is what you get when you purchase Sweet'n Low or Hermesetas. Saccharin is 300 times sweeter than sucrose (table sugar), but has a metallic aftertaste. At one point in the 1970s, saccharin was also thought to cause cancer, but this link was never proven.

In the 1980s, aspartame was invented; it is sold as Nutra-Sweet. It was considered a nutritive sweetener because it was derived from natural sources (two amino acids, aspartic acid and phenylalanine), which means that aspartame is digested and metabolized the same way other protein foods are. Every gram of aspartame has four calories, but because aspartame is 200 times sweeter than sugar, you don't need very much of it to achieve the desired sweetness. In at least 90 countries, aspartame is found in more than 150 product categories, including breakfast cereals, beverages, desserts, candy and gum, syrups, salad dressings, and various snack foods. Here's where it gets confusing: Aspartame is also available as a tabletop sweetener under the brand names Equal and, most recently, PROSWEET. An interesting point about aspartame is that it's not recommended for baking or any other recipe where heat is required. The two amino acids in it separate with heat and the product loses its sweetness. That's not to say it's harmful if heated, but your recipe won't turn out.

For the moment, aspartame is considered safe for everybody, including people with diabetes, pregnant women, and children. The only people who are cautioned against consuming it are those with a rare hereditary disease known as phenylketonuria (PKU), because aspartame contains phenylalanine, which people with PKU cannot tolerate.

Another common tabletop sweetener is sucralose, sold as Splenda. Splenda is a white crystalline powder actually made

Acceptable Daily Intake for Sweeteners	
Sweetener	Intake based on mg/kg body weight
Aspartame	40
Ace-K	15
Cyclamate	11
Saccharin	5
Sucralose	15

Source: Canadian Diabetes Association, "Guidelines for the Nutritional Management of Diabetes Mellitus in the New Millennium. A Position Statement." Reprinted from *Canadian Journal Diabetes Care* 23 (3): 56–69.

Table 1.4

from sugar itself. It's 600 times sweeter than table sugar, but it is not broken down in your digestive system, so it has no calories at all. Splenda can also be used in hot or cold foods and is found in hot and cold beverages, frozen foods, baked goods, and other packaged foods.

In the United States, you can still purchase cyclamate, a non-nutritive sweetener sold under the brand name Sucaryl or Sugar Twin. Cyclamate is also the sweetener used in many weight-control products and is 30 times sweeter than table sugar, with no aftertaste. Cyclamate is fine for hot or cold foods.

The Newest Sweeteners

The newest addition to the sweetener industry is acesuflame potassium (Ace-K), which was approved by the FDA in the late 1990s. About 200 times sweeter than table sugar, Ace-K is sold as Sunett and is found in beverages, fruit spreads, baked goods, dessert bases, tabletop sweeteners, hard candies, chewing gum, and breath fresheners. Although no specific studies on Ace-K and diabetes have been done, the only people who are cautioned against ingesting Ace-K are those on a potassium-restricted diet or people who are allergic to sulpha drugs.

Researchers at the University of Maryland have discovered another sweetener that can be specifically designed for people with diabetes. This sweetener would be based on D-tagatose, a hexose sugar found naturally in yogurt, cheese, and sterilized milk. The beauty of this ingredient is that D-tagatose has no effect on insulin levels or blood sugar levels in people both with and without diabetes. Experts believe that D-tagatose delays the absorption of carbohydrates.

D-tagatose looks identical to fructose and has about 92 percent of the sweetness of sucrose, but only 25 percent of it will be metabolized. Currently, D-tagatose is being developed as a bulk sweetener. As of this writing, it is a few years away from being marketed and sold as a brand-name sweetener.

Stevia

Stevia is a natural, non-fattening sweetener that is 30 to 100 times sweeter than sugar and without any of the aftertaste that is common in many sugar substitutes. It is an herb that has been used in Paraguay and Brazil as a natural sweetener for centuries. It is declared safe to use Japan and is commonly found in soy sauce, chewing gum, and mouthwash. Stevia also is high in chromium (a mineral that helps to regulate blood sugar); is a high source of manganese, potassium, selenium, silicon, sodium, and vitamin A; and contains iron, niacin, phosphorus, riboflavin, thiamine, vitamin C, and zinc.

There has been an explosion of interest in stevia because it is a natural alternative to sugar that contains many nutrients to boot. Stevia is not approved as a sweetener by the U.S. FDA; instead it is legal only as a "dietary supplement." It also remains unapproved as a "food additive" in the United States. Please consult with your diabetes educator about the safety of stevia in your meal planning.

Sugar alcohols

Not to be confused with alcoholic beverages, sugar alcohols are nutritive sweeteners, like regular sugar. They are found naturally in fruits or are manufactured from carbohydrates. Sorbitol, mannitol, xylitol, maltitol, maltitol syrup, lactitol, isomalt, and hydrogenated starch hydrolysates are all sugar alcohols. In your body, these types of sugars are absorbed lower down in the digestive tract and will cause gastrointestinal symptoms if you use too much of them. Because sugar alcohols are absorbed more slowly, they were once touted as ideal for people with diabetes, but because they are a carbohydrate, they still increase your blood sugar just as regular sugar does. Now that artificial sweeteners are on the market in abundance, the only real advantage of sugar alcohols is that they don't cause cavities. The bacteria in your mouth don't like sugar alcohols as much as real sugar.

According to the FDA, even foods that contain sugar alcohols can be labeled "sugar-free." Sugar alcohol products can also be labelled "does not promote tooth decay," which is often confused with "low-calorie."

The Importance of Fiber in Blood Sugar Control

Soluble fiber helps delay glucose from being absorbed into your bloodstream, which not only improves blood sugar control but helps to control post-meal peaks in blood sugar, which stimulates the pancreas to produce more insulin. Fiber in the form of all colors of vegetables will also ensure that you're getting the right mix of nutrients. Experts suggest that you have different colors of vegetables daily—for example, carrots, beets, and spinach. An easy way to remember what nutrients are in which vegetable is to remember that all green vegetables are for cellular repair; the darker the green, the more nutrients the vegetable contains. All red, orange, and purplish vegetables contain antioxidants (vitamins A, C, and E), which boost the immune system and fight off toxins. Studies suggest that vitamin C, for example, is crucial for people with Type 2 diabetes because it helps to prevent complications, as well as rid the body of sorbitol, which can increase blood sugar. Another study suggests that vitamin E helped to prevent heart disease in people with Type 2 diabetes by lowering levels of "bad" cholesterol, but this isn't yet conclusive. Other minerals, such as zinc and copper, are essential for wound healing. The recommendation is to eat all colors of vegetables in ample amounts to get your vitamins, minerals, and dietary fiber. It makes sense when you understand diabetes as a disease of starvation. In starvation, there are naturally lower levels of nutrients in your body that can only be replenished through excellent sources of food.

Soluble vs. Insoluble Fiber

Soluble and insoluble fiber do differ, but they are equally good things. Soluble fiber—somehow—lowers the "bad" cholesterol, or LDL, in your body. Experts aren't entirely sure how soluble fiber works its magic, but one popular theory is that it gets mixed into the bile the liver secretes and forms a type of gel that traps the building blocks of cholesterol, thus lowering your LDL levels. It's akin to a spider web trapping smaller insects. Sources of soluble fiber include oats or oat bran, legumes (dried beans and peas), some seeds, carrots, oranges, bananas, and other fruits. Soybeans are also high sources of soluble fiber. Studies show that people with very high cholesterol have the most to gain by eating soybeans. Soybean is also a *phytoestrogen* (plant estrogen) that is believed to lower the risks of estrogen-related cancers (for example, breast cancer), as well as lower the incidence of estrogen-loss symptoms associated with menopause.

Whole-grain breads are also good sources of insoluble fiber (flax bread is particularly good, because flaxseeds are a source of soluble fiber, too). The problem is understanding what is truly "whole grain." For example, there is an assumption that because bread is dark or brown, it's more nutritious; this isn't so. In fact, many brown breads are simply enriched white breads dyed with molasses. ("Enriched" means that nutrients lost during processing have been replaced.) High-fiber pita breads and bagels are available, but you have to search for them.

What's in a Grain?

Most of us will turn to grains and cereals to boost our fiber intake, which experts recommend should be at about 25 to 35 grams per day. Use the following chart to help gauge whether you're getting enough insoluble fiber. If you're a little under par, an easy way to boost your fiber intake is to simply add pure wheat bran to your foods. Wheat bran is available in health food stores or supermarkets in a sort of "saw dust" form. Three tablespoons of wheat bran equal 4.4 grams of fiber. Sprinkle one to two tablespoons onto cereals, rice, pasta, or meat dishes. You can also sprinkle it into orange juice or low-fat yogurt. It has virtually no calories, but it's important to drink a glass of water with your wheat bran, as well a glass of water after you've finished your wheat bran-enriched meal.

Cereals	Grams of fiber
(based on ½ cup unless otherwise specified)	
Fiber First	15.0
Fiber One	12.8
All Bran	10.0
Oatmeal (1 cup)	5.0
Raisin Bran (¾ cup)	4.6
Bran Flakes (1 cup)	4.4
Shreddies (⅔ cup)	2.7
Cheerios (1 cup)	2.2
Corn Flakes (1¼ cup)	0.8
Special K (1¼ cup)	0.4
Rice Krispies (1¼ cup)	0.3

Breads	Grams of fiber
(based on 1 slice)	
Rye	2.0
Pumpernickel	2.0
12-grain	1.7
100-percent whole wheat	1.3
Raisin	1.0
Cracked-wheat	1.0
White	0

Keep in mind that some of the newer high-fiber breads on the market today have up to seven grams of fiber per slice. This chart is based on what is normally found in typical grocery stores.

Fruits and Veggies

Another easy way of boosting fiber content is to know how much fiber your fruits and vegetables pack per serving. All fruits, beans (a.k.a. legumes), and vegetables listed here show measurements for insoluble fiber, which is not only good for colon health, but also for your heart. Some of these numbers may surprise you!

Fruit	Grams of fiber
Raspberries (¾ cup)	6.4
Strawberries (1 cup)	4.0
Blackberries (½ cup)	3.9
Orange (1)	3.0
Apple (1)	2.0
Pear (½ medium)	2.0
Grapefruit (½ cup)	1.1
Kiwi (1)	1.0

Beans	Grams of fiber
(based on ½ cup unless otherwise specified)	
Green beans (1 cup)	4.0
White beans	3.6
Kidney beans	3.3
Pinto beans	3.3
Lima beans	3.2

Vegetables	Grams of fiber
(based on ½ cup unless otherwise specified)	
Baked potato with skin (1 large)	4.0
Acorn squash	3.8
Peas	3.0
Creamed, canned corn	2.7
Brussels sprouts	2.3
Asparagus (¾ cup)	2.3
Corn kernels	2.1
Zucchini	1.4
Carrots (cooked)	1.2
Broccoli	1.1

Water and fiber

How many people do you know who say: "But I *do* eat tons of fiber, and I'm still constipated!"? Probably quite a few. The reason they remain constipated in spite of their high-fiber diet is because they are not drinking *water* with fiber. Water means water. Milk, coffee, tea, soft drinks, or juice is not a substitute for water. Unless you drink water with your fiber, the fiber will not "bulk up" in your colon to create the nice, soft bowel movements you so desire. Think of fiber as a sponge. Obviously, a dry sponge won't work. You must soak it with water in order for it to be useful. Same thing here. Fiber without water is as useful as a dry sponge. *You gotta soak your fiber!* So here is the fiber/water recipe:

✦ Drink two glasses of water with your fiber. This means having a glass of water with whatever you're eating. (Even if what you're eating does not contain much fiber, drinking water with your meal is a good habit to get into!)

✦ Drink two glasses of water after you eat.

There are, of course, other reasons to drink lots of water throughout the day. For example, some studies show that dehydration can lead to mood swings and depression. Women are often advised from numerous health and beauty experts to drink eight to 10 glasses of water per day for other reasons; water helps you to lose weight; have well-hydrated, beautiful skin; and urinate regularly, which is important for bladder form and function. (Women, in particular, can suffer from bladder infections and urinary incontinence due to diabetes.) By drinking water with your fiber, you'll be able to get up to that "eight glasses of water per day" in no time.

To Treat Low Blood Sugar

If you start to feel symptoms of hypoglycemia, stop what you're doing (especially if it's active) and have some sugar. Next, test your blood sugar to see what it reads. Regular food will usually do the trick. If your blood sugar is below 70 mg/dl (3.8 mmol/L), ingest some glucose. Real fruit juice is better when your blood sugar is low. The best way to get your levels back up to normal is to ingest simple sugar—that is, sugar that gets into your bloodstream fast. Half a cup of any fruit juice or ⅓ of a can of a sugary soft drink is a good source of simple sugar. Artificially sweetened soft drinks are useless. *Your drink must have real sugar.* If you don't have fruit juice or soft drinks handy, here are some other sources high in simple sugar:

+ Two to three tablets of commercial dextrose, sold in pharmacies. If you're taking acarbose or combining it with an oral hypoglycemic agent or insulin, the only sugar you can have is dextrose (Dextrosol or Monoject), due to the rate of absorption.

+ Three to five hard candies (that's equal to about six Life Savers).

+ Two teaspoons of white or brown sugar (or two sugar cubes).

✦ One tablespoon of honey.

Once you've ingested enough simple sugar, your hypoglycemic symptoms should disappear within 10 to 15 minutes. Test your blood sugar 10 minutes after having your sugar to see if your blood sugar levels are coming back up. If your symptoms don't go away, have more simple sugars until they do.

To prevent low blood sugar or hypoglycemia, keep a snack pack with you for emergencies or for unplanned physical activity. The pack should contain:

✦ Juice (two to three boxes or cans).

✦ Sweet soft drinks (sweetened with real sugar, not sugar substitutes; 2 cans).

✦ A bag of hard candies.

✦ Some protein and carbohydrates (packaged cheese/crackers).

✦ Granola bars (great for after exercise).

Vitamins and Minerals

A balanced diet with a variety of nutrients is key when managing Type 2 diabetes. This section is a primer on your vitamin and mineral ABCs.

Chromium

If you have Type 2 diabetes, chromium is considered a valuable trace mineral that helps your body use insulin more effectively; it also benefits the entire circulatory system. Natural medicine practitioners use chromium to help maintain blood sugar levels, reduce arterial plaque, reduce cholesterol, curb sugar cravings, and even help with fat loss. Many people with Type 2 diabetes take chromium supplements and find a dramatic improvement in blood sugar control. In fact, natural medicine practitioners view Type 2 diabetes as a sign that one is deficient in chromium. It is also very useful for people who suffer from hypoglycema. Natural sources of chromium include black pepper, brewer's yeast cheese, clams, corn oil, calves liver, chicken, lean meat, whole-grain cereals, and thyme. (Also see Appendix A.) Chromium supplements range from 25 to 200 micrograms daily for adults, but do not begin this supplement without consulting first with your diabetes practitioner. Many people with Type 2 diabetes combine chromium with vanadium (discussed next) to manage their blood sugar levels without the use of other medications or insulin.

Vanadium

Also a trace mineral, vanadium is said to copy the biological action of insulin, which means it helps your body use insulin more effectively. It is stored in our fat, liver, kidneys, and bones, and its biologically active form is vanadyl sulfate. Vanadium can be used to control blood sugar levels for people with Type 2 diabetes and, used with chromium, can become an alternative therapy under the supervision of a diabetes practitioner. The action of vanadium is blocked by tobacco, so if you smoke this mineral cannot be utilized by the body. Natural sources of vanadium are black pepper, dill seeds, olives, radishes, and whole grains. Vanadium also aids bones and teeth and lowers cholesterol. Vanadium should not be taken as a supplement; instead Vandyl sulfate, the absorbable, biologically active form, can be used solely under the supervision of a doctor. High levels of vanadium can be toxic, and it is not recommended if you are taking lithium for any reason.

FLOWER POWER

Essential oils, comprised from plants (mostly herbs and flowers), can do wonders to relieve stress naturally; many essential oils are known for their calming and antidepressant effects. The easiest way to use essential oils is in a warm bath. Simply drop a few drops of the oil into the bath, and sit and relax in it for about 10 minutes. The oils can also be inhaled (put a few drops in a bowl of hot water, lean over with a towel over your head, and breathe); diffused (using a lamp ring or a ceramic diffuser, that thing that looks like a fondue pot); or sprayed into the air as a mist. You can also rub the oils onto the soles of your feet (where the largest pores are), which will get them working fast!

If you have Type 2 diabetes, the following essential oils are reported to help normalize blood sugar levels: coriander, cypress, dill (supports pancreas functioning and helps normalize insulin levels), eucalyptus, fennel (helps support pancreas), geranium (helps support pancreas), ginger, hyssop, juniper, lavender, rosemary, ylang-ylang, and cinnamon (helps support pancreas).

How to Move

Exercise is essential for maintaining blood sugar levels and managing both Type 1 and Type 2 diabetes. Activity levels have to be carefully balanced with meal plans, because your muscles require sugar to function properly. Chapter 2 discusses activities that help promote cardiovascular health. Chapter 3 discusses hands-on healing techniques that help promote circulation, which can aid with neuropathy. But when it comes to controlling blood sugar, stress reduction is key; stress increases blood sugar levels as well as blood pressure, which can predispose you to cardiovascular complications. (See Chapter 2.) So before you plan to get active, learn how to slow your body down first.

Deep-Breathing Exercises to Relieve Stress

Deep breathing helps to relieve a range of stress-related symptoms such as anxiety, panic attacks, and irritability. In fact, sighing and yawning are signs that that you're not getting enough oxygen in your body; the sigh or yawn is your body's way of righting the situation. Deep breathing calms the nervous system, relaxes the small arteries, and permanently lowers blood pressure. The following deep breathing techniques are modeled after yogic breathing exercises:

Abdominal Breathing: Lie down on a mat or on your bed. Take slow, deep, rhythmic breaths through your nose. When your abdominal cavity is expanded, it means the your lungs have filled completely, which is important. Then, slowly exhale completely, watching your abdomen collapse again. Repeat six to 10 times. Practice this morning and night.

Extended Abdominal Breathing: This is a variation on the previous exercise. When your abdomen expands with air, try three more short inhalations. It's akin to adding those last drops of gas in your tank when your tank is full. Then, when you exhale in one long breath, don't inhale yet. Take three more short exhales.

Abdominal Lift: Stand with feet at about shoulder width, bend the knees slightly, bend forward, exhale completely, and brace your hands above the knees. Then lift the abdomen upward while holding your exhalation. Your abdomen should look concave. Stand erect again and inhale just before you feel the urge to gasp. (Greer Childers, in her video "Body Flex," demonstrates this technique very well.)

Rapid Abdominal Breathing: This is abdominal breathing done at a fast speed so it feels as though your inhalations and exhalations are forceful and powerful. Try this for 25 to 100 repetitions. Each breath should last only a second or so, compared to the 10 to 20 seconds involved in regular deep abdominal breathing.

Alternate Nostril Breathing: Hold one nostril closed, inhaling and exhaling deeply. Then alternate nostrils. This is often done prior to meditation. This is thought to balance the left and right sides of the brain.

Meditate for Stress-Relief

Meditation simply requires you to STOP THINKING (about your life, problems, and so on) and JUST BE. To do this, people usually find a relaxing spot or sit quietly and breathe deeply for a few minutes. Going for a nature walk, playing golf, listening to music, reading inspiring poetry or prose, gardening, listening to silence, and listening only to the sounds of your own breathing are all forms of meditation. These are just a few activities that can be meditative:

+ Taking a walk or hike.
+ Swimming.
+ Running or jogging.
+ Gardening.
+ Golfing.
+ Music appreciation (listening, dancing, and so on).
+ Reading for pleasure.
+ Walking your dog.
+ Practicing breathing exercises.
+ Practicing stretching exercises.
+ Practicing Yoga or Qi gong.

Stretch to Relieve Stress

Stretching improves muscle blood flow, oxygen flow, and digestion. The natural desire to stretch is there for those reasons. The following stretches will help relieve stress and improve tranquility:

+ While sitting or standing, raise your arms above your head. Keep your shoulders relaxed and breathe deeply for five seconds. Release and repeat five times.

+ Gently raise your shoulders in an exaggerated "shrug." Breathe deeply and hold for 10 seconds. Relax, and repeat three times.

+ Sit cross-legged on the floor with spine straight and neck aligned. Focus on your breath, letting it gently fill the diaphragm and the back of the rib cage. On the inhalation, say "so" and on the exhalation, say "hum." Voicing the breath in this manner will keep you focused and relaxed. Continue with "so-hum" until you feel at ease. (This is the Lotus position.)

✦ Sit on your heels. Bring your forehead to the floor in front of you. Breathe into the back of the ribcage, feeling the stretch in your spine. Hold as long as it's comfortable.

✦ Stand tall and find a point across the room at which to focus your gaze. Place the heel of one foot on the opposite inner thigh. Float your arms upward until your palms are touching. Breathe deeply, and hold for five seconds. Release and repeat on the other side.

✦ Lie on your back with palms facing upward, feet turned gently outwards. Focus on the movement of breath throughout your body.

✦ Lie on your belly, with arms at your sides. Bend your legs at the knees and bring your heels in towards your buttocks. Reach back and take hold of the right, then the left ankle. Flex your feet if you're having a hard time maintaining this position. Inhale, raising the upper body as far off the floor as possible. Lift your head, completing the arch. Your knees should remain as close together as possible (tying them together might help here). Breathe deeply and hold for 10 to 15 seconds.

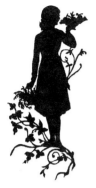

CHAPTER TWO

Preventing Heart Attack and Stroke

What people don't understand is that when the terms *heart disease* or *cardiovascular disease* are used, they refer to your risk of not just heart attack, but also stroke. This chapter explains what happens in heart attack and stroke, as well as the warning signs. It then outlines a drug-free prevention plan you can follow using diet, exercise, and herbal and nutritional supplements. Cardiovascular disease (which leads to heart attack and/or stroke) is certainly the most common disease caused by macrovascular or large blood vessel complications. But most of the other notorious diabetes complications (eye disease, kidney problems, impotence, foot problems, and so on) result when restricted blood flow from macrovascular complications results in nerve damage, known as diabetic neuropathy (which is discussed in Chapter 3).

Understanding Heart Attack

A heart attack is clinically known as a myocardial infarction (MI). The myocardium is the clinical name for the heart muscle. An MI occurs when there is not enough, or any, blood supply to the myocardium, something that happens when one of the coronary arteries is blocked. A coronary artery supplies blood to the heart muscle. Roughly 90 percent of heart attacks are due to a blood clot. A variety of symptoms can occur during a heart attack. *Men have different symptoms than women.*

Heart disease is currently the number-one cause of death in postmenopausal women; more women die of heart disease than of lung cancer or breast cancer. Half of all North Americans who die from heart attacks each year are women.

One of the reasons for such high death rates from heart attacks among women is medical ignorance: Most studies looking at heart disease excluded women (refer to the Introduction), which led to a myth that more men than women die of heart disease. The truth is that more men die of heart attacks before age 50, but more women die of heart attacks after age 50, as a direct result of estrogen loss. Moreover, women who have had oopherectomies (removal of the ovaries) prior to natural menopause increase their risk of a heart attack by *eight times*. Because more women work outside the home than ever before, a number of experts cite stress as a huge contributing factor to increased rates of heart disease in women.

Another problem is that women have different symptoms than men when it comes to heart disease, and so the "typical" warning signs we know about in men—angina, or chest pains—are often never present in women. In fact, chest pains in women are almost never related to heart disease. For women, the symptoms of heart disease (and even an actual heart attack), can be much more vague, seemingly unrelated to heart problems. Signs of heart disease in women include some surprising symptoms, some of which are the same as in men, but some that are completely different:

✦ Shortness of breath and/or fatigue.

✦ Jaw pain (often masked by arthritis and joint pain).

✦ Pain in the back of the neck (often masked by arthritis or joint pain).

✦ Pain down the right or left arm.

✦ Back pain (often masked by arthritis and joint pain).

✦ Sweating (also have your thyroid checked; this is a classic sign of an overactive thyroid gland; also test your blood sugar as you may be low).

✦ Fainting.

✦ Palpitations (ladies, again, have your thyroid checked, also a classic symptom of an overactive thyroid).

✦ Bloating (after menopause, this is a sign of coronary artery blockage).

✦ Heartburn, belching, or other gastrointestinal pain (often a sign of an actual heart attack in women).

✦ Chest "heaviness" between the breasts. (This is how women experience chest pain. Some describe it as a "sinking feeling" or burning sensation; an aching, throbbing, or squeezing sensation; a "hot poker stab between the chest"; or feeling like your heart jumps into your throat.)

✦ Sudden swings in blood sugar.

✦ Vomiting.

✦ Confusion.

Clearly, there are lots of other causes for the symptoms on this list, including low blood sugar. But it's important that your doctor includes heart disease as a possible cause, rather than dismissing it because your symptoms are not "male" (which your doctor may refer to as "typical"). Bear in mind that if you're suffering from nerve damage, you may not feel a lot of these symptoms. Therefore, you should take extra care to be suspicious of anything that feels out of the ordinary.

If you're diagnosed with heart disease, the "cure" is prevention through diet and exercise; protection through hormone replacement therapy is now controversial.

If you are premenopausal and if you have diabetes that is not well controlled, the high blood sugar will cancel out the protective effects of estrogen against heart disease, even if your ovaries are still making estrogen. Therefore, stay alert to the symptoms listed previously. Keeping your blood sugar levels in the normal range (see Chapter 1) will help to restore estrogen's protective properties.

Recovering From a Heart Attack

You can recover from a heart attack, but the damage resulting from the heart attack greatly depends on how long the blood supply to the heart muscle was cut off. The longer the blood supply is cut off, the more damage you will suffer. We all know that a heart attack is a major cause of death, but it can also leave you with varying degrees of disability, depending upon the severity of the attack. For example, roughly half of all heart attack survivors will continue to have heart-related problems, which include reduced blood flow to the heart, called ischemia, and chest pains. As a result, the lifestyle you once enjoyed will need to change: Your diet will need to be restricted to a "heart-smart" diet, and you will need to find ways to reduce lifestyle stress and incorporate more activity into your routine. If you don't make these changes, the risk of repeated heart attacks will loom, which can greatly affect your quality of life. You may also feel more fatigued and winded after normal activities when recovering from a heart attack. Successful recovery greatly depends on the severity of the attack and on lifestyle changes you make after the episode. The same medical strategies designed to prevent a first heart attack can also be used to avoid recurrent episodes.

Understanding Stroke

As mentioned earlier, cardiovascular disease puts you at risk for not just a heart attack, but also a "brain attack" or stroke, which occurs when a blood clot (a clog in your blood vessels) travels to your brain and stops the flow of blood and oxygen carried to the nerve cells in that area. When that happens, cells may die or vital functions controlled by the brain can be temporarily or permanently damaged. Bleeding or a rupture from the affected blood vessel can lead to a very serious situation that could include death. People with Type 2 diabetes are two to three times more likely to suffer from a stroke than people without diabetes. About 80 percent of strokes are caused by the blockage of an artery in the neck or brain, known as an "ischemic stroke"; the remainder are caused by a burst blood vessel in the brain that causes bleeding into or around the brain.

Since the 1960s, the death rate from strokes has dropped by 50 percent. This drop is largely due to public-awareness campaigns regarding diet and lifestyle modification (quitting smoking, eating low-fat foods, and exercising). There are also complimentary healing systems, herbal and nutritional supplements that can reduce stroke incidence.

Strokes can be mild, moderate, severe, or fatal. Mild strokes may affect speech or movement for a short period of time only; many people recover from mild strokes without any permanent damage. Moderate or severe strokes may result in loss of speech and memory and paralysis; many people learn to speak again and learn to function with partial paralysis. How well you recover depends on how much damage was done.

A considerable amount of research points to stress as a risk factor for stroke. (See the section "Natural Ways to Reduce Stress" in Chapter 1 for more.)

Signs of Stroke

If you can recognize the key warning signs of a stroke, it can make a difference in preventing a major stroke or reducing the severity of a stroke.

Call 911 or get to the emergency room if you *suddenly* notice one or more of the following symptoms:

✦ Weakness, numbness, and/or tingling in your face, arms, or legs, especially on one side of the body; this may last only a few moments.

✦ Loss of speech or difficulty understanding somebody else's speech; this may last only a short time.

✦ Confusion.

✦ Severe headaches that feel different from any headache you've had before.

✦ Feeling unsteady, falling a lot.

✦ Trouble seeing in one or both eyes.

If you have any of the signs of stroke just listed, it's important to get to the hospital as soon as possible. There are treatments that can reduce the severity of the damage caused by the stroke, making the difference between partial or severe disability and full recovery.

Common Disabilities Caused by Stroke

There's no question that stroke is responsible for a range of functional and physical disabilities, especially in people older than 45. Depending on the severity of the stroke, your general health, and the rehabilitation process involved, the following impairments may dramatically improve over time:

✧ Weakness or paralysis on one side of the body. This may affect the whole side or just the arm or leg. The weakness or paralysis is always on the opposite side of the body from where the stroke occurred. So if the stroke affected the right side of the brain, you will experience the weakness or paralysis on the left side of your body. Paralysis may affect the face, an arm, a leg, or the entire side of the body. Walking, grasping objects, and the ability to swallow can be affected by one-sided paralysis.

✧ Muscle spasms or stiffness.

✧ Problems with balance and/or coordination.

✧ Problems understanding, speaking, and writing in your first language (called aphasia). This is a common problem, affecting about 25 percent of stroke survivors. At least one-fourth of all stroke survivors experience language impairments. It can take two forms: problems comprehending others or problems articulating their own words. Stroke survivors may be able to think clearly but are unable to make the words "come out right," resulting in disconnected gibberish when they try to speak. The most severe form of aphasia is called global aphasia, which results in the loss of all language abilities: People experiencing global aphasia are not able to understand or communicate in any language. There is also a form of very mild aphasia, called anomic aphasia, where language is mostly unaffected, except for a few words that may be forgotten selectively, such as names of people or particular kinds of objects.

✧ Pain, numbness, or odd sensations (called paresthesia). Pain can be the result of damage to the nervous system (neuropathic pain). Stroke survivors who have a paralyzed arm, for example, may feel as though the pain is radiating outward from the shoulder (the lack of movement causes the joint to be fixed or "frozen"). Physical therapy can help to alleviate this. Pain can also result from a confused signal from the damaged brain, sending out pain to the side of the body that is not affected.

✧ The inability to respond to bodily sensations on one side of the body (called bodily neglect). This means that the ability to feel, touch, and sense pain or temperature can be lost. There may be no recognition of the person's own limb; an arm or leg may not be "noticeable" any more.

✧ Difficulty remembering, thinking, focusing, or learning. Extremely short attention spans, combined with short-term memory loss, can make it difficult for stroke survivors to learn new tasks, make plans, or engage in a complex discussion. Often the ability to connect a thought to an action is lost.

✧ Unawareness of the stroke's effects. A stroke survivor may be paralyzed on one side but not acknowledge the paralysis and have no awareness of the impairment or the fact that a stroke has taken place.

✧ Difficulty swallowing (called dysphagia).

✧ Urinary or bowel incontinence. The ability to sense bladder or bowel urge may be lost, or simply the mobility required to go to the bathroom may be the obstacle. Incontinence becomes less severe with time. Physical therapists can help stroke survivors strengthen their pelvic muscles through special exercises. And by following a timed voiding schedule, incontinence may be solved. In other cases, people can learn to use catheters to prevent other incontinence-related health problems from developing.

✧ Fatigue.

✧ Depression. A mild depression can become a major depression when the stroke survivor loses all engagement and interest in life, loses weight, isn't sleeping properly, and is showing other physical manifestations. Sometimes intervention with antidepressants is necessary if counselling is not effective due to language difficulties.

✧ Mood swings. Natural feelings of anger, anxiety, and frustration can cause extreme mood swings or even personality changes in stroke survivors. Anger is frequently taken out on loved ones, family, or friends.

Recovering From Stroke

According to the National Stroke Association in the Unites States, 40 percent of all stroke survivors experience moderate to severe impairments that require special care; 10 percent will need to be placed in a facility or nursing home; 25 percent have only minor disabilities that enable them to care for themselves; 10 percent will survive the stroke and completely recover with no long-term side effects. The remaining 15 percent of stroke sufferers die shortly after the stroke. Of all stroke survivors, regardless of their level of recovery, 14 percent will have another stroke.

The crucial part of stroke rehabilitation is timing: Rehabilitation should begin as soon as a stroke survivor is stable, which is often within 24 to 48 hours after a stroke. Preventing another stroke involves the same strategies as preventing a heart attack. Obesity, inactivity, and especially smoking spell "ANOTHER STROKE" unless you make some lifestyle changes. You're also at greater risk for another stroke if you have:

✦ High blood pressure (hypertension).

✦ Restricted blood flow (ischemia).

✦ Heart disease.

✦ Celebrated your 65th birthday.

✦ High cholesterol.

Preventing Heart Attack and Stroke (a.k.a. Cardiovascular Disease)

Smoking, high blood pressure, high blood sugar, and high cholesterol (called the "catastrophic quartet" by one diabetes specialist) will greatly increase your risk of heart disease. The way to prevent heart disease and peripheral vascular disease is to modify your lifestyle and eliminate these contributing risk factors. Increasing aerobic activity that helps to strengthen your heart muscle is the next step. Finally, incorporating "heart-healthy" supplements through diet and herbs will make a difference.

Quitting Smoking

You've no doubt been bombarded with information about the health consequences of smoking. But many of you probably don't realize this alarming, yet underreported fact: *The number-one killer of women is cigarettes and smoking.* Smoking-related diseases directly kill more women than any other health or social problem. And yet it remains legal. The number-one killer of women is smoking-related lung cancer; next come smoking-related heart disease, smoking-related stroke, and smoking-related chronic lung diseases, which are very common, yet underreported. And did you know that early menopause and osteoporosis are more common amongst smokers? A single cigarette affects your body within seconds, increasing heart rate, blood pressure, and the demand for oxygen. The greater the demand for oxygen (because of constricted blood vessels and carbon monoxide, a by-product of cigarettes), the greater the risk of heart disease. Lesser-known long-term effects of smoking include a lowering of HDL, or "good" cholesterol, and damage to the lining of blood vessel walls, which paves the way for a host of diabetes complications.

Therapists who specialize in smoking cessation programs for women report that women refer to cigarettes as their "best friend" and will mourn the loss of the cigarettes when they try to quit. The cigarette is a reward for women. The smoking break is seen as "earned" by hard work or stress. Replacing the reward with something else that fills the psychological and spiritual needs is imperative before women can successfully quit. When women seek out specific smoking cessation counseling while trying to quit, the smoking success rate triples. (The tobacco companies ought to pay for this counseling!)

Smoking cessation strategies include:

+ *Herbal and homeopathic smoking cessation aids.* There are many herbal and homeopathic smoking cessation products available. Some use plant sources to reduce cravings; some work by using natural substances to help you "detox."

+ *Behavioral counseling.* Behavioral counseling, either group or individual, can raise the rate of abstinence to 20 to 25 percent. This approach to smoking cessation aims to change the mental processes of smoking, reinforce the benefits of non-smoking, and teach skills to help the smoker avoid the urge to smoke.

+ *Nicotine gum.* Nicotine gum (Nicorette) is now available over the counter. It helps you quit smoking by reducing nicotine cravings and withdrawal symptoms. Nicotine gum helps you wean yourself from nicotine by allowing you to gradually decrease the dosage until you stop using it altogether, a process that usually takes about 12 weeks. The only disadvantage with this method is that it caters to the oral and addictive aspects of smoking (that is, rewarding the "urge" to smoke with a dose of nicotine).

✦ *Nicotine patch.* Transdermal nicotine or the patch (Habitrol, Nicoderm, Nicotrol) doubles abstinence rates in former smokers. Most brands are now available over the counter. Each morning, a new patch is applied to a different area of dry, clean, hairless skin and left on for the day. Some patches are designed to be worn a full 24 hours. However, the constant supply of nicotine to the bloodstream sometimes causes very vivid or disturbing dreams. You can also expect to feel a mild itching, burning, or tingling at the site of the patch when it is first applied. The nicotine patch works best when it is worn for at least seven to 12 weeks, with a gradual decrease in strength (nicotine). Many smokers find it effective because it allows them to tackle the psychological addiction to smoking before they are forced to deal with physical symptoms of withdrawal.

✦ *Nicotine inhaler.* The nicotine inhaler (Nicotrol Inhaler) delivers nicotine orally via inhalation from a plastic tube. Its success rate is about 28 percent, similar to that of nicotine gum. It's available by prescription only in the United States and has yet to make its debut in Canada. As does nicotine gum, the inhaler mimics smoking behavior by responding to each craving or "urge" to smoke, a feature that has both advantages and disadvantages to the smoker who wants to get over the physical symptoms of withdrawal. The nicotine inhaler should be used for a period of 12 weeks.

✦ *Nicotine nasal spray.* The nasal spray reduces craving and withdrawal symptoms, allowing smokers to cut back gradually. One squirt delivers about one mg nicotine. In three clinical trials involving 730 patients, 31 to 35 percent were not smoking at six months. This compares to an average of 12 to 15 percent of smokers who were able to quit unaided. The nasal spray has a couple of advantages over the gum and the patch: Nicotine is rapidly absorbed across the nasal membranes, providing a kick that is more like the real thing, and the prompt onset of action, plus a flexible dosing schedule, benefits heavier smokers. Because the nicotine reaches your bloodstream so quickly, nasal sprays do have a greater potential for addiction than the slower-acting gum and patch. Nasal sprays are not yet available for use in Canada.

✦ *Alternative therapies.* Hypnosis, meditation, and acupuncture have helped some smokers quit. In the cases of hypnosis and meditation, sessions may be private or part of a group smoking-cessation program.

Lowering Blood Pressure Naturally

What is blood pressure? The blood flows from the heart into the arteries (blood vessels), pressing against the artery walls. The simplest way to explain this is to think about a liquid-soap dispenser. When you want soap, you need to pump it out by pressing down on the little dispenser pump, the "heart" of the dispenser. The liquid soap is the "blood" and the little tube, through which the soap flows, is the "artery." The pressure that's exerted on the wall of the tube is therefore the "blood pressure."

When the tube is hollow and clean, you needn't pump very hard to get the soap; it comes out easily. But when the tubing in your dispenser gets narrower as a result of old, hardened, gunky liquid soap blocking the tube, you have to pump much harder to get any soap, and the force the soap exerts against the tube is increased. Obviously, this is a simplistic explanation of a very complex problem, but essentially, the narrowing of the arteries forces your heart to work harder to pump the blood. If this goes on too long, your heart muscle enlarges and becomes weaker, which can lead to a heart attack. Higher pressure can also weaken the walls of your blood vessels, which can cause a stroke.

The term *hypertension* refers to the tension or force exerted on your artery walls. (Hyper means *too much,* as in too much tension.) Blood pressure is measured in two readings: X over Y. The X is the systolic pressure, which is the pressure that occurs during the heart's contraction. The Y is the diastolic pressure, which is the pressure that occurs when the heart rests between contractions. In liquid soap terms, the systolic pressure occurs when you press the pump down; the diastolic pressure occurs when you release your hand from the pump and allow it to rise back to its resting position.

In the general population, target blood pressure readings are less than 130 over 85 (<130/85). Readings greater than 130/85 are considered by diabetes educators to be too high for people with diabetes, but in the general population readings of 140/90 or higher are generally considered borderline, although for some people this is still considered a normal reading. For the general population, 140/90 is "lecture time," when your doctor will begin to counsel you about dietary and lifestyle habits. If they reach 160/100, many people are prescribed a hypertensive drug, which is designed to lower blood pressure.

You can lower blood pressure naturally through stress-reduction techniques, which also help to regulate blood sugar (see Chapter 1). You can also lower blood pressure through diet (see "What to Eat" later in this chapter). Meditation (see Chapter 1) and other forms of hands-on healing (see Chapter 3) also have been shown to improve the condition. Finally, several herbs and supplements have been shown to lower blood pressure (see "Flower Power" later in this chapter).

Lowering Cholesterol Naturally

If you're older than 30, cholesterol levels of less than 5.2 mmol/L (201 mg/dl) are considered healthy. If your cholesterol levels are between 5.2 and 6.2 mmol/L, (201 mg/dl and 240 mg/dl), discuss lifestyle changes with your doctor that can lower cholesterol levels. If your levels are greater than 6.2 mmol/L (240 mg/dl), your doctor may recommend cholesterol-lowering drugs if lifestyle changes were not successful.

For people 18 to 29 years of age, a cholesterol level less than 4.7 mmol/L (182 mg/dl) is considered healthy; a level ranging between 4.7 and 5.7 mmol/L (182 mg/dl and 201) is considered too high, warranting some lifestyle and dietary changes. In this age group, a reading greater than 5.7 (220 mg/dl) may even warrant cholesterol-lowering drugs.

High cholesterol is also called hypercholesterolemia. Another term used in conjunction with high cholesterol is hyperlipidemia, which refers to an elevation of lipids (fats) in the bloodstream; lipids include cholesterol and triglycerides (the most common form of fat from food sources in our bodies). For adults, a triglyceride level less than 2.3 mmol/L (89 mg/dl) is considered healthy.

Total blood cholesterol levels are guidelines only. You also have to look at the relative proportion of high-density lipoprotein (HDL)—or "good" cholesterol—to low-density lipoprotein (LDL) level—or "bad" cholesterol—in the blood. If you're older than 30, an LDL reading of less than 3.4 mmol/L (131.4 mg/dl) and an HDL reading of more than 0.9 mmol/L (34.8 mg/dl) are considered healthy; if you're ages 18 to 29, an LDL reading of less than 3.0 mmol/L (116 mg/dl) and an HDL reading of more than 0.9 (34.8 mg/dl) are considered healthy. Lowering cholesterol is done through diet modification and exercise. (See "What to Eat" and "How to Move" later in this chapter.)

Reducing Stress

There's no question about it: Stress can lead to cardiovascular disease. By employing some of the stress-reduction techniques outlined in chapter 1, you can greatly reduce your risk of heart attack or stroke—the first or second time around.

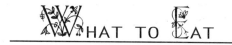

WHAT TO EAT

The most dramatic prevention of cardiovascular disease starts with diet.

Understanding Fat

Fat is technically known as *fatty acids*, which are crucial nutrients for our cells. We cannot live without fatty acids, or fat. If you looked at each fat molecule carefully, you'd find three different kinds of fatty acids on it: saturated (solid), monounsaturated (less solid, with the exception of olive and peanut oils), and polyunsaturated (liquid). When you see the term *unsaturated fat,* it refers to either monounsaturated or polyunsaturated fats.

These three fatty acids combine with glycerol to make what are chemically known as triglycerides. Each fat molecule is a link chain made up of glycerol, carbon atoms, and hydrogen atoms. The more hydrogen atoms that are on that chain, the more saturated or solid the fat. The liver breaks down fat molecules by secreting bile (stored in the gallbladder)—its sole function. The liver also makes cholesterol. Too much saturated fat may cause your liver to overproduce cholesterol. The triglycerides in your bloodstream will rise, perpetuating the problem.

Fat is therefore a good thing—in moderation. As with all good things, though, most of us want too much of it. Excess dietary fat is by far the most damaging element in the Western diet. A gram of fat contains twice the calories as the same amount of protein or carbohydrate. Decreasing the fat in your diet and replacing it with more grain products, vegetables, and fruit is the best way to lower your risk of colon cancer and cardiovascular diseases. Fat in the diet comes from meats, dairy products, and vegetable oils. Other sources of fat include coconuts (60 percent fat), peanuts (78 percent fat), and avocados (82 percent fat). There are different kinds of fatty acids in these sources of fats: saturated, monounsaturated, and polyunsaturated (which, again, is what is meant by the term *unsaturated fat*). Then there is a fourth kind of fat in our diets: trans-fatty acids. (This is a factory-made fat that is found in margarines, for example, which I discuss later on.) To cut through all this big, fat jargon, you can boil down fat into two categories: harmful fats and helpful fats, which the popular press often defines as good fats and bad fats.

Harmful Fats

The following are harmful fats because they can increase your risk of cardiovascular problems, as well as many cancers, including colon and breast cancers. These are fats that are fine in moderation, but harmful in excess (and harmless if not eaten at all):

◆ *Saturated fats.* These are solid at room temperature and stimulate cholesterol production in your body. In fact, the way that saturated fat looks prior to ingesting it is the way it will look when it lines your arteries. Foods high in saturated fat include processed meat, fatty meat, lard, butter, margarine, solid vegetable shortening, and chocolate and tropical oils (coconut oil is more than 90 percent saturated). Saturated fat should be consumed only in very low amounts.

✦ *Trans-fatty acids.* These are factory-made fats that behave just like saturated fat in your body. Foods include animal fats (meat or dairy products) and hydrogenated oils, such as margarine.

Helpful Fats

These are fats that are beneficial to your health and actually protect against certain health problems, including heart disease. These are fats that you are encouraged to use more, rather than less, frequently in your diet. In fact, nutritionists suggest that you substitute harmful fats with these:

✦ *Unsaturated fat.* This is partially solid or liquid at room temperature. The more liquid the fat, the more polyunsaturated it is, which, in fact, *lowers* your cholesterol levels. This group of fats includes monounsaturated fats and polyunsaturated fats. Sources of unsaturated fats include vegetable oils (canola, safflower, sunflower, corn) and seeds and nuts. Unsaturated fats come from plants, with the exception of tropical oils, such as coconut.

✦ *Fish fats (a.k.a. Omega-3 Oils).* The fats naturally present in fish that swim in cold waters, known as omega-3 fatty acids or fish oils, are all polyunsaturated. Again, polyunsaturated fats are good for you: They lower cholesterol levels, are crucial for brain tissue, and protect against heart disease. Look for cold-water fish such as mackerel, albacore tuna, salmon, and sardines.

Factory-Made Fats

An assortment of factory-made fats have been introduced into our diet, courtesy of food producers who are trying to give us the taste of fat without all the calories of saturated fats. Unfortunately, man-made fats offer their own bag of horrors.

That's because when a fat is made in a factory, it becomes a trans-fatty acid, a harmful fat that *not only* raises the level of "bad" cholesterol (LDL, short for low-density lipids) in your bloodstream, but that also lowers the amount of "good" cholesterol (HDL, short for high-density lipids) that's already there.

How, exactly, does a trans-fatty acid come into being? Trans-fatty acids are what you get when you make a liquid oil, such as corn oil, into a more solid or spreadable substance, such as margarine. Trans-fatty acids, you might say, are "the road to hell, paved with good intentions." Someone, way back when, thought that if you could take the good fat—unsaturated fat—and solidify it, so it could double as butter or lard, you could eat the same things without missing the spreadable fat. That sounds like a great idea. Unfortunately, to make an unsaturated liquid fat more solid, you have to add hydrogen to its molecules. This is known as *hydrogenation*, the process that converts liquid fat to semi-solid fat. That ever-popular chocolate bar ingredient "hydrogenated palm oil" is a classic example of a trans-fatty acid. Hydrogenation also prolongs the shelf life of a fat, such as polyunsaturated fat, which can oxidize when exposed to air, causing rancid odors or flavors. Deep-frying oils used in the restaurant trade are generally hydrogenated.

What's wrong with trans-fatty acid?

Trans-fatty acid is sold as a polyunsaturated or monounsaturated fat with a line of advertising copy such as "made from polyunsaturated vegetable oil." Except in your body, it is treated as a *saturated* fat. So really, trans-fatty acids are a saturated fat in disguise. The advertiser may, in fact, say that the product contains "no saturated fat" or is "healthier" than the comparable animal or tropical oil product with saturated fat. So be careful out there: READ YOUR LABELS. The magic word you're looking for is "hydrogenated." If the product lists a variety of unsaturated fats (monounsaturated X oil, polyunsaturated Y oil, and so on), keep reading. If the word hydrogenated appears, count that product as a saturated fat; your body will!

Margarine vs. butter

There's an old tongue twister: "Betty Botter bought some butter that made the batter bitter, so Betty Botter bought more butter that made the batter better." Are we making our batters bitter or better with margarine? It depends.

Since the news of trans-fatty acids broke in the late 1980s, margarine manufacturers began to offer some less "bitter" margarines; some contain no hydrogenated oils, others much smaller amounts. Margarines with less than 60 percent to 80 percent oil (nine to 11 grams of fat) will contain one to three grams of trans-fatty acids per serving, compared to butter, which is 53 percent saturated fat. You might say it's a choice between a bad fat and a *worse* fat.

It's also possible for a liquid vegetable oil to retain a high concentration of unsaturated fat when it's been partially hydrogenated. In this case, your body will metabolize this as some saturated fat and some unsaturated fat.

Nutrition experts advise that you should consume roughly 50 to 55 percent carbohydrates, 15 to 20 percent protein, and less than 30 percent fat daily for a healthy diet. By making the following "swaps" you can significantly lower your dietary fat:

Swap	For
Hamburgers	Veggie Burgers or chicken breast sandwiches
Ground beef	Ground turkey or tofu (soy bean)
Butter	Yogurt, hummus, or reduced-fat margarine
Homogenized milk	Skim or 1% milk
Soft drinks	Club soda or water

Here are some other ways to trim the fat:

✦ Whenever you refrigerate animal fat (as in soups, stews, or curry dishes), skim the fat from the top before reheating and reserving. A gravy skimmer will also help skim fats; the spout pours from the bottom, which helps the oils and fats to coagulate on top.

✦ Powdered non-fat milk is in vogue again; it's high in calcium, low in fat. Substitute it for any recipe calling for milk or cream.

✦ Dig out fruit recipes for dessert. Dishes such as sorbet with low-fat yogurt topping can be elegant. Remember that fruit must be planned for in a diabetes meal plan.

✦ Season low-fat foods well. That way, you won't miss the flavor fat adds.

✦ Lower-fat protein comes from vegetable sources (whole grains and bean products); higher fat proteins come from animal sources.

The following tips apply to preparing meat:

✦ Broil, grill, or boil meat instead of frying, baking, or roasting it. (If you drain fat and cook in water, baking/roasting should be fine.)

✦ Trim off all visible fat from meat before and after cooking.

✦ Adding flour, breadcrumbs, or other coatings to lean meat adds calories, and hence fat.

✦ Try substituting red meat with low-fat turkey meat.

Learning to read the fat content in milk is also a good way to cut down. Consider the following:

✦ Whole milk is made up of 48 percent calories from fat.

✦ 2% milk gets 37 percent of its calories from fat.

✦ 1% milk gets 26 percent of its calories from fat.

✦ Skim milk is completely fat-free.

✦ Cheese gets 50 percent of its calories from fat (unless it's skim milk cheese).

✦ Butter gets 95 percent of its calories from fat.

✦ Yogurt gets 15 percent of its calories from fat.

A Word about Chocolate

A study commissioned by the International Cocoa Organization (ICCO) from findings by the U.S.–based International Cocoa Research and Education Foundation, announced at a news conference during the 2000 global cocoa talks in London, showed that cocoa could possibly cut the risk of developing cancer and heart disease. Apparently cocoa, packed with antioxidants, is filled with compounds that have potentially beneficial human health benefits. Antioxidants have also been found to help prevent plaque sticking to artery walls. The health benefits of cocoa, although still debateable, would be most present in dark, less-processed chocolate as opposed to the candy bars typically sold in stores.

Cut Down on Carbs

Fat is not the only thing that can make you fat. *What about carbohydrates?* Review the sections on understanding carbs and understanding sugar in Chapter 1. It's important to remember that a diet high in carbohydrates can also make you fat. That's because carbohydrates—meaning starchy stuff, such as rice, pasta, breads, and potatoes—can be stored as fat when eaten in excess.

Alcohol

Alcohol delivers about seven calories per gram or 150 calories per drink. It's the sugar in that alcoholic beverage that can also pack in more calories. That said, alcohol has been proven to raise your "good" cholesterol (HDL). This fact was discovered in the late 1980s when researchers probed why France, with all its rich food, had such low rates of heart disease. It was the wine; red wine, in particular, was shown to decrease the risk of cardiovascular disease. Any alcohol will do this, so it's okay to have this stuff, as long as you drink it in moderation.

Dry wines have no added sugar, although they have calories. The same thing goes for cognac, brandy, and dry sherry.

Wine is the result of natural sugar in fruits or fruit juices fermenting. Fermentation means that natural sugar is converted into alcohol. On the other hand, a sweet wine means that it contains some sugar (the amount depends on how sweet the wine is). Dessert wines or ice wines are really sweet; they contain about 15 percent sugar or 10 grams of sugar per two-ounce serving. Sweet liqueurs are 35 percent sugar.

A glass of dry wine with your meal adds about 100 calories. Half–soda water and half-wine (a spritzer) contains half the calories. When you cook with wine, the alcohol evaporates, leaving only the flavor.

If you're a beer drinker, you're basically having some water, barley, and a couple of teaspoons of malt sugar (maltose) when you have a bottle of beer. The barley ferments into mostly alcohol and some maltose. Calorie-wise, that's about 150 calories per bottle plus three teaspoons of malt sugar. A light beer has fewer calories but contains at least 100 calories per bottle.

The stiffer the drink, the fatter it gets. Hard liquors such as scotch, rye, gin, and rum are made out of cereal grains; vodka, the Russian staple, is made out of potatoes. In this case, the grains ferment into alcohol. Hard liquor averages about 40 percent alcohol but has no sugar. Nevertheless, you're looking at about 100 calories per small shot glass, as long as you don't add fruit juice, tomato or clamato juice, or sugary soft drinks.

To Lower Blood Pressure

✦ Limit your salt intake to about 7.5 mL (1½ tsp.) per day by cutting out all foods high in sodium, such as canned soups, pickles, soy sauce, and so on. Some canned soups contain 1,000 mg of sodium, for example. That's a lot!

✦ Increase your intake of calcium or dairy products and potassium (found in, for example, bananas). Some still-unproven studies suggest that people with hypertension are calcium- and potassium-deficient.

Vitamins and Minerals

The following vitamins and minerals are essential to heart health. (See Appendix A for food sources.) Supplements of all of the following are widely available:

✦ The B vitamins (B_{12}, B_6, and so forth).

✦ Vitamin C.

✦ Vitamin E.

✦ Lycopene (a cousin of beta carotene; helps protect against heart disease; found in red fruits and veggies: tomatoes, pink grapefruit, watermelon, guava, and apricots).

✦ Niacin.

✦ Magnesium.

FLOWER POWER

Herbs that are good for the heart are also good for the uterus, incidentally. Plants that strengthen the heart and uterus are either green or red, such as hawthorn, rose, strawberry, raspberry, and motherwort. If you're experiencing perimenopause, you can use these herbs to help reduce hot flashes or night sweats, which can trigger heart palpitations. Drinking lots of water, mineral-rich herbal infusions, or fresh grape juice or eating grapes will help you retain fluids and reduce palpitations as well.

To Nourish/Tone the Heart

+ Wheat germ oil. One or more tablespoons/15 ml daily.

+ Vitamin E oil. One or more tablespoons daily.

+ Flax seed (*Linum usitatissimum*), also known as linseed. Considered the best heart oil—but only if it is absolutely fresh and taken uncooked. One to three teaspoons/five to 15 ml of flaxseed oil first thing in the morning is recommended. You can also grind the seeds and sprinkle them on cereals or salads. You can also soak flax seeds in water and drink first thing in the morning.

+ Other heart protective oils can be found in the fresh pressed oils of borage seed or black currant seed.

+ Other essential fatty acids can be found in plantain, lamb's quarter, or amaranth.

+ Hawthorn berry tincture. Use 25 to 40 drops of the berry tincture up to four times a day. Expect results no sooner than six to eight weeks.

+ Seaweed.

✦ Carotene-rich foods. Look for bright-colored fruits and vegetables. The richer the color, the richer they are in carotene.

✦ Garlic, knoblauch (*Allium sativum*). Greatest heart benefits come from eating it raw, but you can also purchase deodorized caplets.

✦ Lemon balm. Steep a handful of fresh leaves in a glass of white wine for an hour or so and drink with dinner. Or make lemon balm vinegar to use on your salads.

✦ Dandelion root tincture. Use 10 to 15 drops with meals.

✦ Ginseng (*Panax quinquefolium*). Chew on the root or use five to 40 drops of tincture.

✦ Motherwort (*Leonurus cardiaca*). Use a tincture of the flowering tops, five to 15 drops several times a day as needed.

To Calm the Heart

✦ Rose flower essence.

✦ Hawthorn (Crataegus). Try 25 to 40 drops up to four times a day. Slow-acting, it requires about a month of use before you see results.

✦ Motherwort tincture. Ten to 20 drops with meals and before bed or 25 to 50 drops for immediate relief.

✦ Valerian root. As a tea or tincture.

✦ Ginger root tea, hot or cold. (May aggravate hot flashes and heavy flows.)

✦ A piece of real licorice root (to slow palpitations).

To Thin the Blood

Blood thinners, such as aspirin, can reduce the incidence of a stroke or heart attack. A daily spoonful of vinegar made from the leaves, buds, and/or flowers of any of the following herbs can give you the same health benefits as aspirin but also help calcium absorption and improve your digestion: (Do not take blood-thinning herbs if you are bleeding heavily or require surgery.)

✦ Alfalfa.

✦ Birch.

✦ Sweet clover.

✦ Bedstraws.

✦ Poplar.

✦ Red clover.

✦ Willow.

✦ Wintergreen.

✦ Black haw (Viburnum). As a tincture, try a 25-drop dose as needed.

To Lower Blood Pressure

✦ Hawthorn. As a tincture, 10 to 20 drops three times daily.

✦ Motherwort. As a tincture, 10 to 20 drops three times daily.

✦ Dandelion root. As a tincture, 10 to 15 drops with meals.

✦ Potassium. Eighty to 85 percent of people who eat six portions of potassium-rich foods daily will reduce their need for blood-pressure-lowering medication by half or more.

✦ Raw garlic. Just half to one clove of raw garlic a day can dramatically reduce your blood pressure. Mince it raw into a variety of dishes, including eggs, rice, or potatoes.

✦ Ginseng.

✦ Seaweed.

How to Move

If you look up the word *aerobic* in the dictionary, what you'll find is the chemistry definition: living in free oxygen. This is certainly correct; we are all aerobes—beings that require oxygen to live. Some bacteria, for example, are anaerobic; they can exist in an environment without oxygen. All that jumping around and fast movement is done to create faster breathing, so we can take more oxygen into our bodies.

Why are we doing this? Because the blood contains *oxygen*! The faster your blood flows, the more oxygen can flow to your organs. But when your healthcare practitioner tells you to exercise or to take up aerobic exercise, he of she isn't referring solely to increasing oxygen but also to exercising the heart muscle. The faster it beats, the better a workout it gets (although you don't want to overwork your heart, either).

An exercise is considered aerobic if it makes your heart beat faster than it normally does. When your heart is beating fast, you'll be breathing hard and sweating and will officially be in your "target zone" or "ideal range" (the kind of phrases that turn many people off).

There are official calculations you can do to find this target range. For example, it's recommended that by subtracting your age from 220, then multiplying that number by 60 percent, you will find your "threshold level"—which means that your heart should be beating X beats per minute for 20 to 30 minutes. If you multiply the number by 75 percent, you will find your "ceiling level"—which means that your heart should not be beating faster than X beats per minute for 20 to 30 minutes. But this is only an example. If you are on heart medications (drugs that slow your heart down, known as beta blockers), you'll want to make sure you discuss what target to aim for with your health professional.

Improving Oxygen Flow

When more oxygen is in our bodies, we burn fat, our breathing improves, our blood pressure improves, and our hearts work better—which benefits our entire body, leading to regularity, for example. Oxygen also lowers triglycerides and cholesterol, increasing our high-density lipoproteins (HDL) or the "good" cholesterol while decreasing our low-density lipoproteins (LDL) or the "bad" cholesterol. This means that your arteries will unclog and you may significantly decrease your risk of heart disease and stroke. More oxygen makes our brains work better, so we feel better. Studies show that depression is decreased when we increase oxygen flow into our bodies. Ancient techniques such as yoga, which specifically improve mental and spiritual well-being, achieve this by combining deep breathing and stretching, which improves oxygen and blood flow to specific parts of the body.

Exercise has been shown to dramatically decrease the incidence of many other diseases, including cancer. Some research suggests that cancer cells tend to thrive in an oxygen-depleted environment. The more oxygen in the bloodstream, the less hospitable you make your body to cancer. In addition, because many cancers are related to fat-soluble toxins, the less fat on your body, the less fat-soluble toxins your body can accumulate.

The only kind of exercise that will burn fat is aerobic exercise, because *oxygen burns fat*. If you were to go to your fridge and pull out some animal fat (chicken skin, red-meat fat, or butter), throw it in the sink, and light it with a match, it would burn. What makes the flame yellow is oxygen; what fuels the fire is the fat. That same process goes on in your body. The oxygen will burn your fat. You increase the oxygen flow in your body through jumping around/increasing your heart rate or employing an established deep-breathing technique.

You can increase the flow of oxygen into your bloodstream without exercising your heart muscle by learning how to breathe deeply through your diaphragm. There are many yoga-like programs and videos available that can teach you this technique, which does not require you to jump around. The benefit is that you would be increasing the oxygen flow into your bloodstream, which is better than doing nothing at all to improve your health and has many health benefits, according to a myriad of wellness practitioners. Deep-breathing exercises can also help to strengthen digestion and keep you regular.

Finding Your Pulse

You have pulse points all over your body. The easiest ones to find are those on your neck, at the base of your thumb, just below your earlobe, and on your wrist. To check your heart rate, look at a watch or clock and begin to count your beats for 15 seconds (if the second hand is on the 12, count until it reach 15). Then multiply by four to get your pulse.

The Borg Rate of Perceived Exertion (RPE)

This is a way to measure exercise intensity without finding your pulse, and, because of its simplicity, is now the recommended method for judging exertion. This Borg "scale," as it's dubbed goes from six to 20. An extremely light activity may rate a 7, for example, whereas a very, very hard activity may rate a 19. What exercise practitioners recommend is that you do a "talk test" to rate your exertion, too. If you can't talk without gasping for air, you may be working too hard. You should be able to carry on a normal conversation throughout your activity. What's crucial to remember about RPE is that it is extremely individual; what one person judges a 7 another may judge a 10.

Suggested Activities

More Intense	Less Intense
Skiing	
Running	Golf
Jogging	Bowling
Stair-Stepping or Stair-Climbing	Badminton
Trampoling	
Jumping rope	Cricket
Fitness walking	Sailing
Race walking	Swimming
Aerobic classes	Strolling
Roller-Skating	Stretching
Ice skating	
Biking	
Weight-bearing exercises	
Tennis	
Swimming	

Note: Certain activities, such as wrestling or weightlifting, are usually short but very intense. As a result, for people with diabetes, intense exercise is not recommended.

Variations on Jogging

✦ After warming up with a 15-minute walk, simply walk quickly with maximum exertion for two minutes, then slow down for one minute. Keep your heart rate up on the downhill portion of a walk or a hike by adding lunges or squats.

✦ Vary the way you walk for coordination and balance. Try lifting your knees as high as you can, as if marching. Alternate with a shuffle. Do a sideways "crab" walk. To strengthen the rarely used muscles of the ankles and feet, walk first on the outsides, then on the insides of your feet. Or practice walking backwards.

✦ Use a curb for a step workout. Or climb stairs two at a time.

Water Workouts

✦ Start by walking in water that's relatively shallow (waist- or chest-deep). Your breathing and heartbeat will determine how hard you are working. Because you'll be moving fairly slowly, pay attention to your body.

✦ For all-over leg toning, take 50 steps forward, 50 steps sideways in crab-like fashion, 50 steps backward, then 50 steps to the other side.

✦ To tone your arms, submerge yourself from the neck down, bringing the arms in and out as if clapping. The water will provide natural resistance.

✦ Deep-water workouts are the most difficult, because every move you make is met with resistance. Wear a flotation vest and run without touching the bottom for optimum exertion and little or no impact.

✦ You may also want to try buoyant ankle cuffs and styrofoam dumbbells or kickboards for full-body conditioning in the water.

CHAPTER THREE

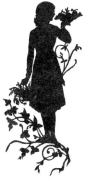

Natural Ways to Get on Your Nerves

Diabetic neuropathy can lead to the loss of nerve function from head to toe and can eventually lead to incontinence and even amputation. This chapter explains exactly what diabetic neuropathy is, how it affects the various parts of your body, and all the natural ways you can prevent nerve damage through diet, exercise, supplements and herbs. (See the "What to Eat," "How to Move," and "Flower Power" sections later in this chapter.)

Understanding Diabetic Neuropathy

When your blood sugar levels are too high for too long, you can develop a condition known as diabetic neuropathy, or nerve disease. Somehow, the cells that make up your nerves are altered in response to high blood sugar. Different groups of nerves are affected by high blood sugar; keeping your blood sugar levels as normal as possible is the best way to prevent many of the following problems. Alternative systems of healing as well as various herbs can aid in preventing or reducing the severity of neuropathy in various parts of the body.

Types of Neuropathy

✦ *Polyneuropathy* is a disease that affects the nerves in your feet and legs. The symptoms are burning, tingling, and numbness in the legs and feet. This is what can lead to amputations in extreme cases. Chapter 8 is devoted solely to foot problems and amputations.

✦ *Autonomic neuropathy* is a disease that affects the nerves you don't notice: the nerves that control your digestive tract (see the gastrointestinal tract section on p. 91), bladder, bowel, blood pressure, sweat glands, overall balance and sexual functioning (see Chapter 7). Addressing each body part individually is covered in the "What to Eat," "How to Move," and "Flower Power" sections.)

✦ *Proximal motor neuropathy* is a disease that affects the nerves that control your muscles. It can lead to weakness and burning sensations in the joints (hands, thighs, and ankles are the most common). These problems can be individually treated with physiotherapy or hands-on healing. When the nerves that control the muscles in the eyes (see Chapter 4) are affected, you may experience problems with your vision, such as double vision. Finally, nerve damage can affect the spine, causing pain and loss of sensation to the back, buttocks, and legs. This can be alleviated through hands-on healing (covered in "How to Move"). Aromatherapy can also work wonders.

Nerve Damage From Head to Toe

What follows is an overview of the body parts most commonly affected by diabetic neuropathy, listed in order from head to toe. Keep in mind that this list is not exhaustive, as there are hundreds of nerve-related problems that can occur. These are the "majors" that affect people with diabetes.

Eyes

For details on all eye and vision problems caused by diabetes, see Chapter 4.

Gastrointestinal Tract (G.I. Tract)

When high blood sugar levels affect your nerve cells, the nerves that control your entire gastrointestinal tract may be affected as well. In fact, 30 to 50 percent of people with diabetes suffer from dysmotility, a condition in which the muscles in the digestive tract become uncoordinated, causing bloating, abdominal pain, and reflux (heartburn).

What is your G.I. tract?

Imagine that your digestive tract is one long subway tunnel with different stops. If you were to look at the G.I. subway map, the first stop is your mouth. The next stop is your pharynx, and the third stop is your esophagus. The esophagus is a major "connecting stop." This is where the train stops for a while before switching tracks and moving on to the more active parts of your gut: the stomach, which connects to your duodenum, which connects to your small intestine, which connects to the last stop on the line, your large intestine.

Swallowing your food triggers all the muscles in your digestive tract to begin contracting in wavelike motions known as peristalsis. The act of swallowing is voluntary, but once the food is down the throat, the rest of the movement through the digestive tract is involuntary, or beyond our control. Our nervous system takes over. The food goes down the throat into the pharynx and into the esophagus. The esophagus connects your throat to your stomach.

In order for your food to get from the esophagus to the stomach, it must go through a crucial tunnel known as the lower esophageal sphincter (LES). When you swallow your food, the LES relaxes to allow your food to pass from the esophagus into the stomach. This is necessary in order to prevent your digested food from backing up into the esophagus.

The stomach is an accordion-like bag of muscle and other tissue near the center of the abdomen, just below the rib cage. The bag expands to accommodate food and shrinks when it is empty. The stomach itself is a holding tank for your food until it can pass through the gastrointestinal tract.

In the same way that the larger coffee grinds stay in the filter, the larger solid particles of food go from the stomach into the duodenum for further digestion, while the mushy, nicely "worked over" food remnants from the stomach will quickly pass from the duodenum into the small intestine (also known as the mid-gut or small bowel). The small intestine is usually called just that, but technically it can be categorized as the duodenum, jejunum, and ileum. For simplicity, most refer to it as the small intestine.

A series of various tubes along your G.I. tract empty food particles from one into the next. This process depends on continuous movement, known as *motility*, which is controlled by nerves, hormones, and muscles. In fact, if you're experiencing problems with other parts of your body, the motility can be slowed down (resulting in constipation and bloatedness) or speeded up (resulting in diarrhea).

By the time your food gets into the small intestine, your food is now mushed up by the digestive secretions of your stomach, pancreas, and biliary tract. All this mush stays in the small intestine for a relatively long period of time, and all the usable nutrients are absorbed through the intestinal walls. These nutrients include digested molecules of food, water, and minerals from the diet. The waste products are sent to the large intestine (the colon or large bowel), where they sit around for about a day or two before they are expelled in the form of stools.

Diabetic nerve disease affects the G.I. tract north of the colon—that is, everything between the esophagus and small intestine. A number of things can go wrong north of the colon, because hundreds of nerves and secretions (hormones, enzymes, and chemicals that help to break down your food into usable nutrients) go to work for us whenever we eat. If even one hormone or enzyme is "off" in your system, there will be consequences. There are upper G.I. disorders and lower G.I. disorders. The upper G.I. disorders, which can be caused by diabetic nerve disease, can include heartburn/reflux, a symptom of a larger problem of dysmotility (see the following section), also known as gastroesophageal reflux disease (GERD). Diabetic nerve disease can also cause problems south of the colon, where muscles controlling the bowel become uncoordinated, causing them to open, leak stool, and allow bacteria to grow abnormally in the colon, resulting in bacterial-related diarrhea. This can be controlled with antibiotics.

Understanding dysmotility

Dysmotility means "things not moving very well." Food travels from your esophagus into your stomach, which slowly releases it into the small intestine. There can be problems on any or all "floors" of this elevator. Things can get stuck between the esophagus and stomach, causing symptoms of heartburn and reflux (see the following section). In this case, the lower esophageal sphincter relaxes when it should be taut, allowing food to come back up. Or things can get stuck between the stomach and small intestine, which causes symptoms of bloating, early fullness, and gas. So when things aren't moving very well, you can have a lot of discomfort. This is known as a motility disorder.

Dysmotility, with all of its varying symptoms, is typically a very chronic condition. Symptoms keep coming back, and by the time dysmotility is finally diagnosed most people have had these symptoms for a long time. The only way you can stop symptoms from recurring is to change certain lifestyle habits (losing weight, quitting smoking, and staying in control of blood sugar levels may improve your condition) or take a motility drug as a "maintenance" drug. If your dysmotility goes on for a long time, it could also lead to inflammation of the esophageal lining, a condition known as esophagitis. This can lead to the narrowing of the esophagus. (When your esophagus is inflamed, it narrows, just the way your shoes are suddenly too tight when your feet expand.)

Understanding heartburn/reflux

As just described, your food must pass from your esophagus into your stomach through the lower esophageal sphincter, which opens and closes through a variety of involuntary muscular contractions. If you have diabetic nerve disease, the sphincter may not shut completely after dumping your ingested food particles into the stomach. So what happens? The food, now bathed in your stomach acid, can actually come back up the sphincter, causing a burning sensation in your chest, and even a spreading pain throughout your neck and arms, which may even be mistaken for a heart attack. You can also experience nausea, belching, and regurgitation of that half-digested food. When it comes back up the sphincter, it doesn't taste as good as it did going down. Thanks to the acid and enzymes it's been exposed to, the food will taste sour and bitter in your throat. The problem will be aggravated when you bend forward or lie down. In fact, you may even find that after an experience such as this, you wake up with a sore throat. This problem is clinically called *acid reflux*, and in lay terms it is known as heartburn or acid indigestion. For the remainder of this book, the term *heartburn/reflux* will be used.

Heartburn/reflux usually lasts about two hours. Most people find that standing up relieves the burning; that's because gravity helps. You could also take an antacid to clear acid out of the esophagus. Not everyone will experience the same degree of heartburn. Heartburn/reflux can be mild, moderate, or severe. It all depends on why it's occurring, how often it occurs, when it occurs, and how much food backup you have. But for the most part, chronic heartburn/reflux is the first sign of a more serious, underlying health problem such as dysmotility or GERD.

A number of atypical, unusual, or "odd" symptoms can suggest you have heartburn/reflux, too. They include:

✦ Morning hoarseness.

✦ Drooling.

✦ Coughing spells.

✦ Waking up with a sore throat.

✦ Asthmalike symptoms (or the worsening of asthma symptoms if you are asthmatic). In these cases, you may be having heartburn/reflux at night, which is obstructing your breathing passages, causing all the strange symptoms from coughing to asthma.

Skin

High blood sugar levels, combined with poor circulation, puts the skin—all over your whole body—at risk for infections ranging from yeast to open-wound-related infections. You may form scar tissue or develop strange yellow pimples (a sign of high fat levels in the blood), boils, or a range of localized infections. Yeast infections, which typically plague women who experience them in the form of vaginal yeast infections, can develop not just in the vagina, but in the mouth (called thrush), under the arms, or wherever there are warm, fatty folds. All skin, whether on the feet or elsewhere, can become dry and cracked, requiring a daily regimen of cleaning, moisturizing, and protecting. (Sexual functioning is discussed in detail in Chapter 7.)

Kidneys

Diabetic kidney disease requires a separate chapter. (For details, please see Chapter 6.)

Gallbladder

The gallbladder stores bile for the liver. But we don't really need the gallbladder, because the liver is large enough to store as much bile as we'd ever want or need anyway. Nevertheless, we do come equipped with this extra storage space. Bile isn't a very reliable product to store because it can form into little stones inside the gallbladder, known as gallstones (or calculi). When your gallbladder isn't emptying properly, a process controlled by nerves and that can be impaired with diabetic nerve disease, you can form gallstones. Symptoms occur when the stones become large enough to obstruct the bile ducts. And when this happens, you are said to have *gallbladder disease*.

The symptoms of a gallbladder attack are quite severe; you'll feel sudden, intense pain in the upper abdominal region (which may shoot into your back), often after a fatty meal (though it may not be related to meals). Vomiting frequently brings relief, although nausea is not a symptom. The pain may then subside over several minutes or hours. Many people mistake gallstone symptoms with heartburn or a heart attack.

The obstruction can become infected or even gangrenous, which is a dire emergency (you don't want gangrene inside your abdominal cavity!). Usually gallbladder disease presents itself as a series of gallbladder "attacks" in which you'll feel the pain after a meal and, if there's infection, may even experience a fever. The attacks will become progressively worse until you decide to have the darned thing removed. As a rule, any abdominal pain accompanied by a fever means there is some sort of serious infection going on in there, which is an emergency, warranting emergency medical attention.

Because of other factors, such as taking estrogen (many women use some form of estrogen product), gallbladder problems are much more common in women than men (one in five women after age 50 versus one in 20 men) and also in women who are on hormone-replacement therapy after menopause, which is now very controversial. Estrogen-containing oral contraceptives are also associated with gallstones.

What to Eat

First, if you smoke, STOP! See page 66 in Chapter 2 for smoking cessation information. Diabetic neuropathy will be aggravated by smoking no matter how vigilant you are about blood sugar control, diet, and exercise.

Meal Planning

It is essential that you stick to your meal plan and check your blood sugar frequently. (See Chapter 1 for more details.)

Cutting Fat

For people who suffer from upper G.I. problems that result from diabetic dysmotility, cutting down on high fat can dramatically improve matters. (For more details, see Chapter 2, which discusses heart-smart diets in detail.)

Cut the Caffeine

Caffeine is hard on the gut, which can aggravate diabetic dysmotility. By cutting it down or out, many people find their upper G.I. symptoms improve. Here's a checklist of how much caffeine some foods contain, with the milligrams of caffeine in parentheses:

Coffee (5-oz. cup)

> Brewed, drip method (60–180)
>
> Brewed, percolator (40–170)
>
> Instant (30–120)
>
> Decaffeinated, brewed (2–5)
>
> Decaffeinated, instant (1–5)

Tea (5-oz. cup)

> Brewed, major brands (20–90)
>
> Brewed, imported brands (25–110)
>
> Instant (25–50)
>
> 12-ounce glass of iced (67–76)

Other

> 6-ounce glass of caffeine-containing soft drink (15–30)
>
> 5-ounce cup of cocoa beverage (2–20)
>
> 8-ounce glass of chocolate milk (2–7)
>
> Single-ounce serving of milk chocolate (1–15)
>
> Single-ounce serving of dark chocolate, semi-sweet (5–35)
>
> Single square of baker's chocolate (26)
>
> Serving of chocolate-flavored syrup (4)

Add the Fiber

You gotta go regularly to feel well *north* of your colon! Fiber is the part of a plant your body can't digest, which comes in the form of both water-soluble fiber (which dissolves in water) and water-insoluble fiber (which does not dissolve in water but, instead, absorbs water); this is what's meant by soluble and insoluble fiber. Soluble and insoluble fiber do differ, but they are equally beneficial. (Because fiber is essential to stabilizing blood sugar, it is discussed at length in Chapter 1.)

Spices Good for Digestion

Coriander: Eases gases and works to tone the digestive system. Use powdered or whole-seed, or garnish with fresh leaves (cilantro).

Cardamom: Reduces the mucus-forming effects of dairy products. Use powdered or whole seeds.

Turmeric: Generally improves metabolism and helps you to digest proteins. Use the root ground. (Gives dishes a yellowish color and can stain clothes and china.)

Black Pepper: Stimulates appetite and helps you digest dairy products. Use freshly ground.

Cumin: Helps reduce gases and generally tones the digestive system. Use seeds whole or powdered.

Fennel: Helps prevent gas. Chew the seeds after eating, or add them to vegetables that tend to produce gas when cooking. Use whole or powdered.

Ginger: Aids digestion and respiration. Also helps to relieve gas, constipation, or indigestion. Use root fresh or dried. (Note: Ginger can aggravate bleeding ulcers.)

Cinnamon: Naturally cleanses your digestive system. Use powdered or in sticks or pieces.

Nutmeg: Helps your body absorb nutrients from food, but should be used sparingly.

Clove: Helps your body absorb nutrients, too. Use whole or ground.

Cayenne: Helps to simulate your digestive juices and is known for having a "cleansing action" within the large intestine. Helps to relieve that feeling of "fullness" after eating a heavy meal.

Vitamins and Minerals

Biotin: Good for muscles and skin. Found in Brewer's yeast, egg yolks, legumes, whole grains, organ meats, and soybeans.

Zinc: Aids in wound-healing. Can be taken as supplement. (See Appendix A for food sources.)

Proline: An amino acid that helps wound-healing and cartilage; also helps the body to make collagen. Found in meat.

Choline: Promotes gallbladder and liver health. Found in Brewer's yeast, fish, legumes, organ meats, soybeans, wheat germ, and lecithin.

FLOWER POWER

- Aconite (known as *Fu tsu* in Chinese healing system). This is considered a warm herb that is most "yang" of all the Chinese herbs. It helps with circulation, heart, nervous system, small intestine, spleen and urinary tract system—almost all of the body parts affected by neuropathy. It can help reduce numbness. It should be taken under the supervision of a traditional Chinese medicine doctor only.

- Tienchi (Chinese herb). Aids in wound-healing.

The following herbs are good for the circulatory system:

Capsicum.

Garlic.

Ginger.

Ginkgo biloba.

Gotu kola.

Hawthorn.

Prickly ash.

To aid with healing cuts and open wound, the following essential oils help (use in a warm bath, see p. 51):

Tea tree oil.

Emu oil (from Australia; also good for moisturizing skin).

Bergamot.

Chamomile.

Clove.

Eucalyptus.

Frankincense.

Juniper.

Lavender.

Myrrh.

Rose.

Rosemary.

Rosewood.

Thyme.

The following scents can improve circulation:

Birch.

Cinnamon bark.

Clary sage.

Cypress.

Hyssop.

Nutmeg.

How to Move

When it comes to neuropathy, the best thing to "move" is what alternative healing systems call the life force energy. This is by far the most important way to improve circulation.

Qi Gong Exercises

Every morning, all over China, people of all ages gather at parks to do their daily qi gong exercises. Pronounced *Ch'i Kung,* these are exercises that help get your life force energy (called the *qi* or *chi* in Chinese) flowing and unblocked (See Chapter 5). Qi gong exercises are modeled after movements in wildlife (such as birds or animals), movement of trees, and other things in nature. The exercises have a continuous flow, rather than the stillness of a posture seen in yoga. Using the hands in various positions to gather in the qi, move the qi, or release the qi is one of the most important aspects of qi gong movements.

One of the first group of qi gong exercises you might learn are the "seasons"—fall, winter, spring, summer, and late summer. (There are five seasons here.) These exercises look akin to a dance with precise, slow movements. The word *qi* means vitality, energy, and life force; the word *gong* means practice, cultivate, and refine. The Chinese believe that practicing qi gong balances the body and improves physical and mental well-being. These exercises push the life force energy into the various meridian pathways that correspond to organs. It is the same map used in pressure-point healing. Qi gong improves oxygen flow and enhances the lymphatic system. Qi gong is similar to tai chi, except that it allows for greater flexibility in routine. The best way to learn qi gong is through a qualified instructor. You can generally find qi gong classes in the alternative healing community. Check health-food stores and other centers that offer classes such as yoga or tai chi. Qi gong is difficult to learn from a book or video.

Acupuncture

Acupuncture is an ancient Chinese healing art that aims to restore the smooth flow of life energy (or qi) in your body. Acupuncturists believe that your qi can be accessed from various points on your body, such as your ear for example. Each point is also associated with a specific organ. Depending on your physical health, then, an acupuncturist will use a fine needle on a very specific point to restore qi to various organs. Each of the roughly 2,000 points on your body has a specific therapeutic effect when stimulated. The National Institute of Health (NIH) is funding research that studies the effects of acupuncture on depression, attention-deficit disorder, hypersensitivity disorder, osteoarthritis, and postoperative dental pain. In one large study, acupuncture offered short-term relief to 50 to 80 percent of patients with acute or chronic pain. It's now believed that acupuncture stimulates the release of endorphins, which is why it's effective in reducing pain. That could help alleviate symptoms associated with neuropathy.

Reflexology

Today's version of an ancient healing and relaxation technique is probably as old or older than acupuncture. Western reflexology was developed by Dr. William Fitzgerald, an American ear, nose, and throat specialist who talked about reflexology as "zone therapy." Reflexology is practiced in several cultures, including Egyptian, Indian, African, Chinese, and Japanese. In the same way as the ears are a map to the organs, with valuable pressure points that stimulate the life force, here the feet play the same role.

In a nutshell, the "sole is qi (the life force) to the soul." By applying pressure to certain parts of the feet, reflexologists can ease pain and tension and restore the body's life force, be it qi in China or prana in India.

Reflexologists don't limit themselves to the feet, however. They will also work on hands and ears, although the feet are the most common site. As with most Eastern healing arts, reflexology aims to release the flow of energy through the body along its various pathways. When this energy is trapped for some reason, illness can result. When the energy is released, the body can begin to heal itself.

A reflexologist views the foot as a microcosm of the entire body. Individual reference points or reflex areas on the foot correspond to all major organs, glands, and parts of body. Applying pressure to a specific area of the foot stimulates the movement of energy to the corresponding body part. To find a good reflexology map that shows you where to work your own pressure points, visit *www.reflexology-usa.net*. This is Dwight D. Byers's Web site. Byers, who uses the famous Ingham Method, is considered the foremost reflexology expert who trains other reflexologists.

Active Living

Gravity helps your food go down. You have to get off your couch and move if you want your G.I. symptoms to improve without drug therapy. See Chapter 2 for more information about incorporating serious exercise into your routine. That said, there are many ways you can adopt an active lifestyle that do not involve exercise per se. Here are some suggestions:

✦ If you drive everywhere, pick the parking space further away from your destination so you can work some daily walking into your life.

✦ If you take public transit everywhere, get off one or two stops early so you can walk the rest of the way to your destination.

✦ Choose stairs more often over escalators or elevators.

✦ Park at one side of the mall and then walk to the other.

✦ Take a stroll after dinner around your neighborhood.

✦ Volunteer to walk the dog.

✦ On weekends, go to the zoo or get out to flea markets, garage sales, and so on.

Other ways to keep active is to choose a sport or activity:

More Intense	Less Intense
Skiing	
Running	Golf
Jogging	Bowling
Stair-Stepping or Stair-Climbing	Badminton
Trampoling	Cricket
Jumping rope	Sailing
Fitness walking	Swimming
Race walking	Strolling
Aerobic classes	Stretching
Roller-Skating	
Ice-Skating	
Biking	
Weight-bearing exercises	
Tennis	
Swimming	

Postures That Improve Digestion

Locust:	Lie on your belly with your arms folded beneath you, palms pressed in to your body. Extend both legs until they lift up and off the floor. Keep the toes pointed. Release.
Cobra (Upward Facing Dog):	Lie on your belly with your palms down and adjacent to your shoulders. Slowly raise your upper body, lifting all but the lower abdomen toward the ceiling. Breathe deeply. Release.
Fish:	Lie on your back. Place your hands under your sitting bones, palms pressed to the floor, feet flexed. Gently roll one, then the other shoulder inward, shortening the distance between your shoulder blades. (Your chest will naturally arch upwards.) Breathe, lengthening your abdominals and ribcage. Release.

Reducing Stress

Experts cite stress as a leading cause of many upper and lower G.I. problems. Your G.I. tract is controlled by your nervous system, which is why it can definitely react when you're under stress. In the same way that you can sweat, blush, or cry under emotional stress, your G.I. tract may also react to stress by "weeping"—that is, producing excessive water and mucus and overreacting to normal stimuli such as eating.

What often happens, however, is that there is a delayed "gut reaction" to stress, and you may not experience your G.I. symptoms until your stress has passed. Apparently, under stress your brain becomes more active as a "defense." (For example, when we're running away from a predator, we have to think quickly and act quickly, so our heart rates increase, we sweat more, and so on). During this defensive mode, the entire nervous system can become exaggerated (that's what causes "butterflies" in the stomach). The nerves controlling the G.I. tract therefore become highly sensitive, which can cause an array of G.I. symptoms that aggravate diabetic dysmotility. (See Chapter 1 for more details on stress reduction.)

CHAPTER FOUR

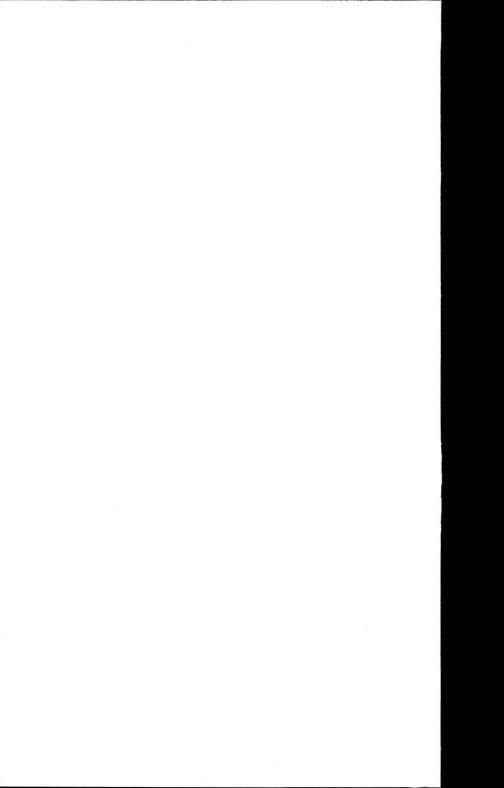

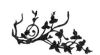

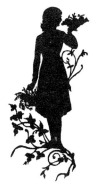

Turning Your
Eyes to Nature

Diabetes is the leading cause of new blindness in adults. Of people with Type 2 diabetes, 78 percent experience diabetes eye disease, clinically known as diabetic retinopathy. Microvascular complications (see Chapter 1) damage the small blood vessels in the eyes. High blood pressure, associated with macrovascular complications (see Chapter 1), also damages the blood vessels in the eyes.

Although 98 percent of people with Type 1 diabetes will experience eye disease within 15 years of being diagnosed, in Type 2 diabetes eye disease is often diagnosed *before* the diabetes. In other words, many people don't realize they have diabetes until their eye doctors ask them if they have been screened for diabetes. In fact, 20 percent of people with Type 2 diabetes already have diabetes eye disease before their diabetes is diagnosed. The longer you've had diabetes, the more at risk you are for diabetes eye disease. Because people are living longer with diabetes, it is now considered the most common cause of blindness under age 65 and the most common cause of new blindness in North America.

Eighty percent of all eye disease is categorized as non-proliferative eye disease, meaning "no new blood-vessel growth" eye disease. This is also called background diabetic eye disease. In this case, the blood vessels in the retina (the part of your eyeball that faces your brain, as opposed to your face) start to deteriorate, bleed or hemorrhage (known as micro-aneurysms), and leak water and protein into the center of the retina (called the macula). This condition is known as macular edema and causes vision loss, which sometimes is only temporary. However, without treatment, more permanent vision loss will occur. Although non-proliferative eye disease rarely leads to total blindness, as many as 20 percent of those with non-proliferative eye disease can become legally blind within five years.

Proliferative eye disease means "new blood-vessel growth" eye disease. In this case, your retina says, "Because all my blood vessels are being damaged, I'm just going to grow *new* blood vessels!" This process is known as neovascularization. The problem is that these new blood vessels are deformed, or abnormal, which makes the problem worse, not better. These deformed blood vessels look a bit like Swiss cheese; they're full of holes and have a bad habit of suddenly bleeding, causing severe damage without warning. They can also lead to scar tissue in the retina, retinal detachments, and glaucoma, greatly increasing the risk of legal blindness.

Diabetes can also cause cataracts, which are a cloudings of the lens inside the eye, which blur vision.

This chapter will cover signs of eye disease and failing vision, visual aids, and coping with low vision or blindness using natural tools in your environment. All of the information in this chapter discusses improving vision without the use of surgery or drugs. But first, the best step is *prevention*.

Preventing Diabetes Eye Disease

The adage "early detection is your best protection" is perhaps no truer than when it comes to diabetes eye disease! *It's crucial to have frequent eye exams*. The average person has an eye exam every five years. You need to see an eye doctor twice a year from now on.

During an eye exam, an ophthalmologist will dilate your pupil with eye drops, then use a special instrument to check for the following:

✦ Tiny red dots (signs of bleeding).

✦ A thick or "milky" retina, with or without yellow clumps or spots (signs of macular edema).

✦ A "bathtub ring" on the retina—that is, a ring shape that surrounds a leakage site on the retina (also a sign of macular edema).

✦ "Cottonwool spots" on the retina—that is, small fluffy white patches in the retina (signs of new blood vessel growth or more advanced eye disease).

Today, it's estimated that if everyone with impaired glucose tolerance (see Chapter 1) went for an eye exam once a year, blindness from diabetes eye disease would drop from 8 percent in this group to 1 percent.

Stop Smoking

Because smoking also damages blood vessels and diabetes eye disease is a blood vessel disease, smoking will certainly aggravate the problem. Quitting smoking may help to reduce eye complications. (See Chapter 2 for more details on smoking cessation.)

Avoid Eye Infections

High blood sugar can predispose you to frequent bacterial infections, including conjunctivitis (commonly known as pink eye). Eye infections can also affect your vision. To prevent eye infections, make sure you wash your hands before you touch your eyes, especially before you handle contact lenses.

Stay in Control

The Diabetes Complication and Control Trial showed that Type 1 patients, who suffer most from diabetes eye disease, were able to delay the onset of eye damage by staying in tight blood sugar control (see Chapter 1). Also, by controlling your blood pressure and cholesterol (see Chapter 2), you can help to reduce the effects of swelling in the central part of the retina.

Signs of Eye Disease

Diabetes eye disease is prevalent in women with Type 1 and Type 2 diabetes. In the early stages of diabetes eye disease, there are no symptoms. That's why you need to have a thorough eye exam every six months. As the eye damage progresses, you may notice blurred vision. The blurred vision is due to changes in the shape of the lens of the eye. During an eye exam, your ophthalmologist may notice yellow spots on your retina, signs that scar tissue has formed on the retina from bleeding. If the disease progresses to the point where new blood vessels have formed, vision problems may be quite severe as a result of spontaneous bleeding or detachment of the retina.

Vision can fail in two areas: central vision and peripheral vision. Central vision is identifying an object in focus. Peripheral vision is seeing out of the corner of your eye. When we lose our central vision, we lose the ability to focus on fine detail: print, television images, details of faces, and so forth. When we lose our peripheral vision, we develop "tunnel vision" (a common sign of glaucoma, for example). This restricts us from seeing obstructions, causing us to bump into corners of chairs and doors and trip on many objects. Diabetes eye disease affects both central and peripheral vision.

Vision loss is often very gradual. It may not be something you notice suddenly. Signs of failing vision are important clues that you may have diabetes eye disease that is progressing. The following are classic signs of failing or deteriorating vision:

+ You sit closer and closer to the television.

+ You squint in order to see.

+ You need a stronger prescription for your glasses or contacts.

+ You have difficulty reading the newspaper.

+ You are bothered by bright lights.

+ You are more accident-prone: bumping into chairs or doors, tripping over curbs and steps, and knocking things over all the time.

+ You can't see well in the dark or at night; night driving is difficult.

All About Visual Aids

If your vision is deteriorating, a range of visual aids are available that can make living and working far easier than it was for many of our parents and grandparents who suffered from partial or complete vision loss. This is, in part, due to a range of technologies that can enhance images through magnification, lighting, and color contrast. A number of tactile products exist, as does using the Braille alphabet.

Visual aids are used by people with partial sight, also known as low vision, reduced vision, or impaired vision. Some people still refer to low vision as being "legally blind" or having partial blindness. These terms are slowly falling out of favor because of myths surrounding what blindness means in most cases (see "Coping With Low Vision or Blindness" later in this chapter). Of the Canadians who identify themselves as visually impaired, fewer than 20 percent are totally blind—that is, without any usable vision. When you hear that "diabetes causes blindness," it is not untrue, but it usually refers to a scenario in which you are visually impaired with *some usable vision left*, which makes you a candidate for visual aids (low-vision aids).

Making Things Larger

One of the most common visual aids involves products that can magnify an image, known as magnification devices. These devices can extend the image over a large enough area of the retina for it to be detected by the healthy cells at the edges, or periphery. Magnification devices typically magnify as much as 22 times the normal size. For example, my computer can magnify my screen so that the words I type are 500 percent larger than they actually are. Magnification aids commonly used can be telescopes, which make distant objects appear closer; binoculars, which many people can use to watch television, movies, or plays; monoculars, which can help you read distance objects, such as street names, house numbers, or bus numbers; or pocket magnifiers, illuminated magnifiers, or stand-mounted magnifiers, which are frequently used for a wide assortment of tasks from working to crafts and leisure activities.

Some people need different visual aids for different tasks. Typically one aid will be used for fine detail tasks, such as reading, another one for watching television, and another one for outdoor use.

You can also buy many items with large print, including large-print books, telephones, and clocks.

High-tech magnification devices

Magnification devices can be either low-tech (as in magnifying reading glasses) or high-tech (as in software or hardware). Generally, the more high-tech the device, the more expensive it is. If you can afford it, here is a sample of some of the higher-tech magnification products that are available. Typically, high-technology products work with existing hardware you may already own, such as desktop or laptop computers, palm devices, and so on. It may be sold as software that works with your equipment or sold as an "interface," a smaller piece of hardware you connect to something such as a computer, which can transform data, manipulate data, and so on.

Many computer companies offer a range of adaptive products. For example, Xerox makes a product called the Reading Edge, which is a transportable reading machine that offers magnification, scanning, a speech synthesizer (if you can't read it, you can hear the data), optical character recognition (allowing you to dictate letters that come out in print), and so on. Another product, called the Reading AdvantEdge, is a software program that can make your home computer do all of these things (except perhaps to scan).

Large-print computer-access products are another kind of high-tech aid that allow you to select a preferred font for the computer's display of characters, change the foreground or background colors of the screen, and display large print as full-screen mode. Almost any word-processing software has some capacity to magnify, but these products, such as MAGic, can magnify the screen image from two through 20 times the normal size. A range of other options to optimize visual image are offered with these various large-print packages.

Closed-circuit television (CCTV) can also help with magnification. This is a system that it is similar to a video camcorder device. Anything you place in front of the camera will be broadcast on your TV screen so that you can see it more closely: Books, recipes, prescriptions, photographs, and so on can all be enhanced with CCTV systems. One product called Magni-Cam, for example, is a handheld electronic magnifier that connects to any television set. The camera weighs only 198 g (seven oz.) and doesn't require any focusing.

There are literally hundreds of high-tech visual aids available. The best way to find them is through the Internet. Go to your favorite software/hardware manufacturer's Web site and search for *adaptive products, products for the visually impaired,* or *visual aids.*

Making Things Brighter

Products that improve lighting are also visual aids. Direct light sources can dramatically improve the ability of people with low vision to complete tasks by reducing glare, improving background light, and so forth. Low-tech solutions involve:

+ A direct light source focused on the task, not on the person.

+ Increasing the light bulb wattage on lamps.

+ Using high-intensity lights that reduce glare but increase light.

+ Retrofitting the home with adjustable indirect track lighting for flexibility.

+ Installing fluorescent lighting under kitchen cabinets and near the sink and stove.

+ Keeping a flashlight by the stove.

+ Equipping the home with night lights to ease the transition from darkness to light.

+ Getting a few floor lamps or other non-glare light sources near the TV.

+ Installing dimmer switches or three-way light bulbs.

+ Sitting with the back to the window to reduce glare (especially in public places).

+ Wearing a hat with a visor for light sensitivity outdoors.

+ Getting ultraviolet-inhibitor sunglasses for outdoor glare. (Ask your optician about this.)

Making Things Stand Out

You can make objects stand out by using color-coding, another type of visual aid. The general rule is to contrast the background with the foreground; smoother textures tend to make colors appear light, whereas uneven surfaces tend to make colors appear darker.

In the home, for example, using color contrast can make it easier to find things or identify objects. You can buy markers that are brightly colored and that dry into a hard plastic (Hi-marks, for example). They can be used to mark appliances, such as the stove, washer, or dryer. Nail polish or colored tape can be used on keys or mailboxes. Brightly colored elastic bands can be used as markers for jars or tins. You can even use colored magnets (such as colored alphabet letters) for metal surfaces. In the kitchen, dark pots against a white stove (or the reverse) can help. Otherwise, you can put colored tape near the end of the pot handles. When you eat, color contrast between placemats or tablecloth and dishes makes it easier to distinguish between them than using table coverings with glossy finishes or patterns. Electrical outlets should also contrast with the surrounding walls; just buy colored wall plates for your outlets.

A little redecorating using color can work wonders. Color-contrasting paint can be used around door frames or to paint cupboards, for example.

Color contrasting can be used to separate your clothes (by color or texture). For the bathroom, you can use colored toothpaste that will contrast with white bristles on the toothbrush; a color-contrasted bath mat will help, as will using a colored soap in the shower or bath. Using different colors for towels and washcloths can help you tell which you're using.

Making Things Touchy-Feely

Tactile products are "touchy-feely." These products are either designed with Braille lettering (the raised dots system invented by Louis Braille in the 19th century and still used today) or clearly tactile in other ways. Essentially, Braille is another way to read and write printed information. It is equivalent, in every way, to print. You can read or write words, numbers, music notations, and any other symbols that appear in print. It works by arranging combinations of the six dots of the Braille "cell." Braille is read by touch and is therefore a tactile language. Most people use the first finger on one or both hands to read it. Braille can be used for any language, mathematics, scientific equations, and computer notations. The only people who can't use Braille are those who suffer from numbness in their fingers or hands, but most people with diabetes-related numbness will feel it in their legs or feet, not their fingers.

You can get hundreds of Braille-adapted products, including glucose meters, pill organizers, thermometers, and so on. Braille is actually all around us in modern architecture, but the sighted population doesn't always notice. For example, most elevators are equipped with Braille lettering on the buttons. There are also Braille computers with Braille keyboards and a refreshable Braille screen. (Braille computers are very expensive, however, with each Braille cell [letter, as in A, B, C, and so on] retailing at roughly $55 per cell.)

In short, the availability of tactile products is not the problem; everything you could possibly need in life either comes in Braille lettering or can probably be specially ordered.

Braille as a second language

The problem with tactile products has more to do with people's reluctance to learn Braille. Most people equate learning Braille with being totally blind, which is truly unfortunate. Braille is just as useful for people who have partial sight and, in many situations, knowing it can make life a little easier. It's akin to knowing a second language to enhance your communications skills. For example, learning Spanish comes in handy in all kinds of situations, from being able to communicate and make friendships with Spanish-speaking people to ordering food in a Mexican restaurant. It's the same thing with Braille: *It comes in handy and can enhance, rather than detract from, your life.*

People who lose their hearing are similarly reluctant to learn sign language (also called signing), but in numerous situations, signing would make a hearing-impaired person's life easier.

When you know a different language, you have access to a new community of people, too, which is very important when you feel isolated or alone. You already know that when you can talk to someone else who has diabetes, you immediately "connect" with one another because you share a common struggle. It's the same thing with vision loss: Meeting someone else who is coping with vision loss helps you feel less alone and allows you to talk to someone who knows what you're going through. Imagine Braille as a bridge to new friends and a new community. Braille can also keep you employed, as it enables you to make notes on documents, read a spreadsheet, take minutes at a meeting, file materials, read diskette labels, and so on.

Braille also lessens your dependency on voice synthesizers (for reading or writing), audiotape recordings, magnifiers, and other print enhancers. These are great visual aids, but they are not convenient in all circumstances. At home, you can also use Braille to label CDs, clothing, spices, cans, and so forth. You can also play games, such as cards, Scrabble, backgammon, and chess.

Making Things Talk

An obvious visual aid is a product that talks. Before the popularity of voice synthesizers, audio-taped books were about the only talking product available. Today, voice synthesizers can be used with almost any information product, including small things such as thermometers. With scanners, you can scan printed material into a voice-synthesized computer that can tell you what something says, including labels or fine print. One danger is an overreliance on voice-synthesized products, however.

Coping With Low Vision or Blindness

The hardest part of losing some or all of your vision is coping with it. This has a lot to do with misconceptions about what "blindness" means. Blindness is defined as total loss of sight. That said, more than 80 percent of people who are considered blind can usually make out the outlines of objects, identify the sources of light, ascertain the direction of light, distinguish light from dark, and so forth.

Registered Blind

There are degrees of blindness that go from low or impaired vision to profound vision loss. All these definitions can be classified as "Registered Blind," a category that allows you to be eligible for income tax and other government benefits. You are considered Registered Blind when you have visual acuity in your better eye, after correction, of 20/200 or less. That means that you can see at 20 feet what someone with perfect vision can see at 200 feet. (Visual acuity refers to the sharpness and clarity of "near vision"—that is, close-up objects.) You can also be Registered Blind if your visual field (peripheral vision) results in a narrowing of your central vision to 20 degrees or less (you may be able to read, but walking around is hazardous because you can't see what's around you).

So that means that most people who are Registered Blind see *something*. A lot of people who appear sighted in public and who seem to get around just fine with some visual aids are Registered Blind.

The white cane is often perceived as an announcement to the world that you are visually impaired, *but that's not necessarily a bad thing.* One of the chief purposes of the cane is to get people to be considerate and *move out of your way* when you are trying to get around. It also gives permission for people to approach you to offer their assistance. For example, as a frequent subway passenger, I have never witnessed a caned individual attempt to get on and off a train without being deluged with offers of assistance. All kinds of people, from a myriad of age groups and backgrounds, offer to help. The offers of assistance also help to reinforce a sense of community for the sighted subway travelers; it's good to see people get involved and offer unsolicited help!

An identification cane is a collapsible white cane that primarily identifies you as visually impaired, but it can also be used for depth perception on stairs or curbs. There is also the white support cane, which says, "I have vision loss, *and* I have trouble walking." This cane is designed to support your weight. Finally, a long cane can be thought of as your "whiskers": a probe that senses things in front of you. It is mostly used in the home or in unfamiliar surroundings. Before you use it, the Canadian Institute for the Blind encourages a training session with an orientation and mobility instructor.

A Word About Denial

Coping with vision loss often involves overcoming denial that you are losing your sight. This is a normal reaction, but it can also foster behaviors that are not helpful in the long run. It can lead to a lesser quality of life, because those in denial often refuse hclp with visual aids. Some people may also become overly dependent on others, which can foster a range of unhealthy relationships with friends or family members. You may rely on family members to cook, clean, shop, and so on for you. Vision loss does *not* have to mean loss of mobility, and, with the right visual aids and training, you can do lots of things on your own and regain your independence.

Coping With Blind Ignorance

The most disabling part of vision loss is the ignorance you encounter from the general public. You may want to pass on the following tips to friends and family members (who, in turn, can tell a few more people), which can make life a little easier for everyone:

✦ When speaking to someone with vision loss, face them and speak clearly in a moderate tone. Don't shout. Vision loss does not mean the person is hearing impaired, too.

✦ Anyone can act as a sighted guide. Just offer your arm and say, "My name is X. Here's my arm if you need some assistance." Then allow the person to take it. Never just grab someone's arm without permission. When acting as a sighted guide, walk at a normal pace. You can hesitate slightly before stepping up or down.

✦ Don't pat a guiding dog, please. And speak to the person, not the dog!

✦ If you're giving directions, use phrases such as "on your left" or "right behind you" instead of "over there" or "over here."

✦ At social gatherings, describe who is in a large group; don't just leave someone alone in the middle of the room with no sense of who's in it.

✦ Identify yourself when you approach a visually impaired guest so that she or he knows who's talking.

Here are some suggestions for dining with a visually impaired person:

✦ Describe what's on the table to illicit a mental image of the food and help enhance appetite.

✦ Describe what's on the plate clockwise to make it easier.

✦ Assist with cutting meat if it's requested.

✦ Use extra large napkins if possible.

WHAT TO EAT

The most important way to prevent vision loss is to stick to your meal plan and test your blood sugar frequently. (Meal plans and blood sugar testing are discussed in Chapter 1.)

Lower Your Blood Pressure and Cholesterol

By controlling your blood pressure and cholesterol (see Chapter 2) through diet and herbal approaches, you can help to reduce the effects of swelling in the central part of the retina.

Vitamins and Minerals

Part of the caratonoid family, lutein is an antioxidant that helps preserve vision and prevent blindness through macular degeneration. Supplement doses recommended are six to 20 mg per day. Lutein can be found in collard greens, corn, kale, mustard greens, and spinach.

FLOWER POWER

The following herbs are known for improving vision:

✦ Bilberry. The active ingredients are anthocyanodieds, which protect small blood vessels and rebuild the light-adapting retinal pigments in the eyes. Available in liquid extracts or capsules.

✦ Eyebright. Specifically helps with cataracts and eye infections.

The following essential oils are known for improving vision when applied to bottoms of feet:

+ Frankincense.

+ Juniper.

+ Lemongrass.

How to Move

Ayervedic techniques for improving eyesight include:

+ Gazing at the rays of the sun at dawn for five minutes each day.

+ Gazing at a steady flame, morning and evening, for ten minutes.

+ Avoiding reading in bed.

Remaining Active With Low Vision

As you know from previous chapters, staying physically active is an important way to manage your diabetes and help to stabilize blood sugar. Visual impairment does not mean you need to be inactive. Swimming, golfing, skiing, curling, tandem bicycling, and walking are just a few of the many activities you can enjoy with a few adaptations. For example, you can utilize a sighted guide to help you with some of these activities. You can incorporate brightly colored guide wires in swimming pools; you can find a sighted partner for tandem cycling (maybe a sighted friend who needs to get active, too, and could use a partner). You can find beeping balls for ball sports or tactile markers for bowling. The range of visual aids or adaptations is endless, and you're encouraged to contact the American Foundation for the Blind (*www.afb.org/*) to discuss how to use adaptations to accommodate your activities. (In Canada, contact the Canadian Institute for the Blind or CNIB; *www.cnib.ca*.)

CHAPTER FIVE

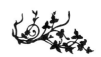

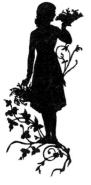

Taking a Bite out of Nature

High blood sugar levels get into your saliva and feed the bacteria in your mouth. The bacteria, in turn, break down the starches and sugars to form acids that eventually break down your tooth enamel. This is how cavities are formed.

Moreover, damage to the small blood vessels in your gums can lead to periodontal problems, and blood sugar levels naturally rise when you're fighting a gum infection (known as a periodontal infection), such as an abscess. Preventing dental problems means the usual regimen (see "Combating Gum Disease" later in this chapter). You're also advised to have your teeth cleaned and examined at least every six months or more depending on your periodontal health and to avoid sugary foods (which you should be doing anyway). Unfortunately, this is just not enough information for most people with diabetes, especially if they already have gum disease.

Gum Disease and Heart Disease

Here is some news you don't want but must have: Gum disease increases your risk of heart disease. The link has been known for years, but very few people are aware of it. It's believed that inflamed gums can produce inflammatory by-products that affect the cardiovascular system. Also, the bacteria that spread in gum disease can produce damage to blood platelets, causing clots. Because people with Type 2 diabetes are already at high risk for heart disease and stroke (see Chapter 2), this means that Type 2 diabetes, combined with gum disease, puts you at extreme risk for heart disease. Treating or preventing gum disease can have a positive effect on your cardiovascular health.

Diabetes-Related Gum Disease

Gum disease, also called periodontitis, is often not noticeable until it's serious. It's caused from bacteria that are normally in the mouth, which can vary in aggressiveness. The bacteria settle around and under the gum line (where the gums and teeth meet); this is called plaque. Brushing and flossing can remove the plaque, preventing it from hardening into tartar (also called calculus). Bacterial infections can develop from tartar. At this stage, it's called gingivitis, but as the bacterial infection worsens, you're looking at full-blown gum disease or periodontitis.

Healthy gums go around the tooth the way a cuff goes around your wrist. When the gums fit more loosely, the bacteria get deeper into the gums, alongside the tooth, near the bone, where no toothbrush or floss can go (but a periodontist can with special cleaning instruments). The bacteria can cause an inflammatory reaction that erodes the bone supporting the teeth, making them loose. Eventually, you may have to have your teeth pulled and wear dentures.

Roughly 90 percent of all North Americans have gum disease at some point in their lives. Because people with diabetes have more frequent infections and are slower to heal due to inefficient white blood cells, this can also affect the gums. Second, any kind of infection, such as a urinary tract infection, or even a cold or a flu, will increase blood sugar levels. So when the gums become infected, it can have serious consequences for your overall health. Also, damage to small vessels (microvascular complication) can affect the support tissues in the gums, too.

Two things are going on with diabetes-related gum disease: High blood sugar can make you vulnerable to gum disease, and gum disease can increase your blood sugar levels even more because it is an active infection. (Of course, the same can be said for any infection, but many of us don't think of gum disease as an active infection.)

The Smoking Gum

If you've read other chapters in this book, you know what a bad combination smoking and diabetes make. Unfortunately, smoking can predispose you to gum disease, making your already-high risk from diabetes higher still. More smokers than non-smokers have gum disease; at least half of all cases of gum disease are directly linked to smoking, and some studies show that as much as 75 percent of gum disease is smoking-related.

If you quit smoking, you can reduce the likelihood of developing gum disease; the longer you've not smoked, the greater the chances you will not suffer gum disease.

Smokers have the highest risk of gum disease, ex-smokers have the next highest, and non-smokers have the lowest risk. Diabetes is another significant risk factor, though, which means if you smoke and have diabetes, you're at highest risk of developing serious gum disease. (See Chapter 2 for information on smoking cessation. Quitting smoking will make it easier for you to treat your gum disease, too.)

Combating Gum Disease

The strategy is to try to prevent gum disease, if possible, by employing all of those boring "dentist" rules that have been drilled into you for as long as you can remember: brushing after eating, flossing, rubber-tip massage, fluoride rinses, and, most of all, frequent checkups. Going for regular cleaning by your dentist or dental hygienist to remove built-up tartar is considered a "first-line" prevention strategy; however, it is what you do at home that can really make the difference. Ask your dentist or hygienist to show you how to brush and floss properly; it's amazing how many of us were taught the wrong way by our parents or dentists of yesteryear, and those poor habits can contribute to dental problems. We also should not be using brushes with hard bristles.

If you have diabetes, consider going for routine dental cleanings every three months instead of every six months. Extra cleaning can really help to reduce plaque, which is the building block of gum disease.

Many years ago, the manufacturers of Close-Up toothpaste used the line "How's your love life?" to sell their toothpaste. Well, they were onto something. *Did you know that gum disease can be transmitted by kissing?* If your lover has gum disease, chances are he or she has aggressive bacteria that can be transferred to your mouth, too. For more information about gum disease transmissibility, it's worth visiting the Web site *www.periotrans.com.*

Signs of Gum Disease

Any of the following are signs that you have gum disease:

✦ *Bleeding gums.* This is often the first sign of gum disease. You may notice bleeding when you brush your teeth or floss. If your gums are bleeding, it's always a sign of gum disease. (You can also have gum disease without having bleeding gums.)

✦ *Receding gums.* This occurs when the gum is not covering as much tooth as it should, sometimes exposing the roots.

✦ *New spaces between teeth.* This is called migration and refers to two teeth that used to "touch" but that no longer do.

✦ *Chronic bad breath (halitosis).* Bad breath can be caused by poor digestion or by insufficient cleaning and a buildup of plaque. Of course, there are also many foods that cause bad breath. But if bad breath persists after proper cleanings and a good oral-hygiene routine (including brushing the tongue), gum disease is probably the reason, where pus and bleeding are contributing to the bad breath problem.

✦ *Red gums.* Healthy gums should be the color of salmon or coral, not blood. If you breathe through your mouth, red gums are more common, too.

✦ *Loose teeth.*

✦ *Less tapered gum "coverage" around the teeth.* The gum should meet the tooth at a knife-edge margin. If this margin is rolled and swollen, it's a sign of gum disease.

✦ *Shiny gums.* Gums should have some "stippling" to them (little dots) so they don't shine; shiny red gums are not a good thing.

When you notice any of these signs of gum disease, see your dentist. Your dentist will look for a host of things you can't see yourself, such as root cavities, pockets in the gums, tooth decay under the gum line, and so on.

What to Do if You Have Gum Disease

If gum disease has progressed beyond the early-stage gingivitis, you'll be referred to a periodontist. This is a dentist who has done a three-year residency in treating gum problems and gum disease. Periodontists can restore gum tissue or regenerate it. At your first visit, the periodontist will use a special probe that can measure gaps between the gums and teeth, as well as look for exposed roots, which need special care, too. Gaps between the gum and teeth are called pockets and normally shouldn't be deeper than one to three millimeters. Pockets deeper than this can be a sign of serious gum disease.

Periodontists may also do special cleanings called root planing, where the gum tissues are usually anaesthetized, and the roots of the teeth (which may be exposed or still covered by gums) are cleaned. The goal is to get rid of as much plaque and tartar as possible to prevent bacterial infections from developing or progressing once they have developed. Root planing may also involve using antibiotics to help kill off the bacteria deep inside the gums. Gum surgery involves restoring the gumline to a more readily cleanable state by reducing the pockets and removing the diseased state.

If you have gum disease, it must be treated. Doing so will lower your blood sugar levels and can improve your overall health and ability to control your diabetes. If gum disease has progressed to the point where your teeth are loose or keep becoming infected (forming root infections, abscesses, and so on), dentures may be the next step. Compared to losing your eyesight (see Chapter 4), a kidney (see Chapter 6), or a foot (see Chapter 8), dentures are certainly not the end of the world. But each set of dentures comes with its own set of problems. For more information on dentures, contact the American Dental Association (*www.ada.org*). If you still have your teeth, the information in this chapter can help you keep them.

WHAT TO EAT

A gum-smart diet can start with the right chewing gum! If you don't have the opportunity to brush after eating, chew some "dental gum," a new product that has exploded onto the shelves—"in the toothpaste section," as one commercial tells us. Dozens of chewing-gum brands have introduced dental gums. These gums may have tartar-fighting or whitening agents, are sugar-free, and so on. When you chew a sugar-free gum after eating, you get the saliva activated, which can wash away bacteria that form plaque.

All that stuff you tell your kids about sugar and cavities applies to adults, too! Use the same rules for yourself. Avoid sticky sweets and sugary snacks (something you need to do anyway if you're managing diabetes and planning meals). Ask your dietitian about "gum-smart" snacks (nuts, seeds, raw fruits and vegetables, and so on).

If you plan to eat something sweet, have it with a meal so your saliva can wash it down. After meals, if you can't brush, rinse your mouth with water and chew some sugar-free or dental gum.

FLOWER POWER

The following essential oils can be used alone, or in combination with sesame oil to massage the gums:

+ Tea tree oil.
+ Myrrh.

How to Move

Moving your hands is the best way to prevent gum disease! Whether you want to prevent gum disease or are being treated for gum disease, brushing and flossing are doing the right thing, but many of us are doing the *right* thing the *wrong* way! The first thing most people do when their gums start to bleed from brushing or flossing is stop. This is the worst response. Keep at it; the bleeding should stop after a few days as you strengthen the gums.

Sometimes people use the wrong brushes. Use soft bristles; hard bristles can damage the gums, and you can "brush off" gum tissue, which can lead to recession and root exposure.

Next, people buy the wrong floss and assume that flossing doesn't "work" for them. If you're finding that your floss is shredding or breaking, get another brand. If your teeth are very close together, finer, unwaxed floss is better. If shredding is a problem, a thicker, waxed floss is better.

I'm all for recycling, but *please* don't recycle your floss. Use a clean piece for each tooth. Take a long piece of floss and inch your way to the end with each tooth. By the way, if the plaque you remove is foul-smelling, that is a sign you have bad breath. You can recheck for the smell when you floss next; if the smell improves, so has your breath, and you can rest assured that it was a plaque problem and not a chronic, unsolvable problem.

Brushing your teeth for five seconds is better than nothing, but the American Dental Association recommends you brush every 24 hours at least for about three minutes. Again, use soft instead of hard brushes. With soft bristles, you can also massage your gums and loosen plaque that is deeper within. Ask your dentist to show you how to do this and for a sample of a special brush you can use for hard-to-reach places; it can brush behind your front teeth, for example, an area often missed, or behind your side teeth.

Cleaning Your Tongue

Bacteria that can wreak havoc on your gums can live on your tongue. Tongue scrapers are now available at most pharmacies, and can also alleviate chronic bad breath (halitosis). In ayervedic medicine, tongue scraping has long been a part of health maintenance, and the scraper, which can "massage" the tongue, can apparently help massage the internal organs that correlate with the different areas of the tongue, according to ayervedic and Chinese medicine.

CHAPTER SIX

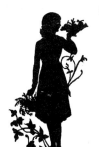

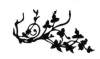

Keeping Your Kidneys

Diabetic kidney disease, also known as diabetic nephropathy, is what happens when macrovascular complications *and* microvascular complications converge. The high blood pressure that is caused by macrovascular complications, combined with the small blood vessel damage caused by microvascular complications, can cause kidney failure—something you *can* die from unless you have dialysis (filtering out the body's waste products through a machine) or a kidney transplant. The majority of people with Type 1 diabetes will face problems with their kidneys; about 15 percent of people with Type 2 diabetes will develop kidney disease, which often goes by the terms *renal disease* or *nephropathy.*

When your kidneys have failed and you require dialysis, this is known as end-stage renal disease (ESRD); diabetes is considered to be the leading cause of kidney disease, responsible for roughly 45 percent of all cases of end-stage renal disease. Put another way, roughly 45 percent of all dialysis patients have diabetes. The good news is that the risk of developing chronic kidney disease increases with the length of time you have had diabetes, so by getting your diabetes under control early in the game, you may be able to prevent kidney disease or kidney failure.

What Do Your Kidneys Do All Day?

Kidneys are the public servants of the body; they're busy little bees! If they go on strike, you lose your water service, garbage pickup, and a few other services you probably don't even appreciate.

Kidneys regulate your body's water levels. When you have too much water, your kidneys remove it by dumping it into a large storage tank, your bladder. The excess water stays there until you're ready to "pee it out." If you don't have enough water in your body (or if you're dehydrated), your kidneys will retain the water for you to keep you balanced.

Kidneys also act as your body's sewage filtration plant. They filter out all the garbage and waste that your body doesn't need and dump it into the bladder; this waste is then excreted into your urine. The two waste products your kidneys regularly dump are *urea* (the waste product of protein) and *creatinine* (waste products produced by the muscles). In people with high blood sugar levels, excess sugar will get sent to the kidneys, and the kidneys will dump it into the bladder, too, causing sugar to appear in the urine.

Kidneys also balance calcium and phosphate in the body, needed to build bones. Kidneys operate two little side businesses on top of all this. They make hormones. One hormone, called renin, helps to regulate blood pressure. Another hormone, called erythropoietin, helps bone marrow make red blood cells.

What Affects Your Kidneys

There are a few things that converge that result in kidney damage.

The Macro Thing

When you suffer from cardiovascular disease, you probably have high blood pressure. High blood pressure damages blood vessels in the kidneys, which interferes with their job performance. As a result, they won't be as efficient at removing waste or excess water from your body. And if you are experiencing poor circulation, which can also cause water retention, the problem is further aggravated.

Poor circulation may cause your kidneys to secrete too much renin, which is normally designed to regulate blood pressure, but in this case increases it. All the extra fluid and the high blood pressure place a heavy burden on your heart—and your kidneys. If this situation isn't brought under control, you'd likely suffer from a heart attack before kidney failure, but kidney failure is inevitable.

The Micro Thing

When high blood sugar levels affect the small blood vessels, it includes the small blood vessels in the kidney's filters (called the nephrons)—hence the term "diabetic nephropathy." In the early stages of nephropathy, good, usable protein is secreted in the urine. That's a sign that the kidneys were unable to distribute usable protein to the body's tissues. (Normally, they would excrete only the waste product of protein—urea—into the urine.)

Another microvascular problem that affects the kidneys is nerve damage. The nerves you use to control your bladder can be affected, causing a sort of sewage backup in your body. The first place that sewage hits is your kidneys. Old urine floating around your kidneys isn't a healthy thing. The kidneys can become damaged as a result, aggravating all the conditions discussed so far in this section.

The Infection Thing

There's a third problem at work here. If you recall, frequent urination is a sign of high blood sugar. That's because your kidneys help to rid the body of too much sugar by dumping it into the bladder. Well, guess what? You're not the only one who likes sugar; bacteria, such as *E. coli* (the "hamburger bacteria"), like it, too. In fact, they thrive on it. So all that sugary urine sitting around in your bladder and passing through your ureters and urethra can cause this bacteria to overgrow, resulting in a urinary tract infection (UTI) such as cystitis (inflammation of the bladder lining). The longer your urethra, the more protection you have from UTIs. Men have long urethras; women have very short urethras, and at the best of times are prone to these infections—especially after a lot of sexual activity, explaining the term "honeymoon cystitis." Sexual intercourse can introduce even more bacteria (from the vagina or rectum) into a woman's urethra due to the close space the vagina and urethra share. Women who wipe from back to front after a bowel movement can also introduce fecal matter into the urethra, causing a UTI.

Any bacterial infection in your bladder area can travel back up to your kidneys, causing infection, inflammation, and a big, general mess, aggravating all the other problems.

The Smoking Thing

In the same way that smoking contributes to eye problems (see Chapter 4), it can also aggravate kidney problems. Smoking causes small vessel damage throughout your body. (See Chapter 2 for information on smoking cessation.)

Signs of Diabetic Kidney Disease

Obviously, there are a lot of different problems going on when it comes to diabetes and kidney disease. If you have any of the following early warning signs of kidney disease, see your doctor as soon as possible:

✦ Bad taste in the mouth (sign of toxins building up; see also Chapter 5 on tooth decay).

✦ Blood or pus in the urine (a sign of a kidney infection).

✦ Burning or difficulty urinating (a sign of a urinary tract infection).

✦ Fever, chills, or vomiting (a sign of *any* infection).

✦ Foamy urine (a sign of kidney infection).

✦ Foul-smelling or cloudy urine (a sign of a urinary tract infection).

✦ Frequent urination (a sign of high blood sugar and/or a urinary tract infection).

✦ High blood pressure (see Chapter 2).

✦ Itching.

✦ Leg swelling or leg cramps (a sign of fluid retention).

✦ Less need for insulin or oral diabetes medications.

✦ Morning sickness, nausea, and vomiting.

✦ Pain in the lower abdomen (a sign of a urinary tract infection).

✦ Protein in the urine (a sign of microvascular problems).

✦ Puffiness around eyes or swelling of hands and feet (a sign of edema, or fluid retention).

✦ Weakness (a sign of anemia).

In the early stages of kidney disease, there are often no symptoms at all. Many of the symptoms just listed are signs that your kidney function has deteriorated to the point where toxins and wastes have built up, causing, for example, nausea and vomiting, fluid retention, even chronic hiccups. Heart failure (not to be confused with a heart attack, discussed in Chapter 2) and fluid in the lungs are characteristic of very late stages of kidney failure.

When you experience any of these symptoms, it's crucial to have a blood test that looks for creatinine levels. Again, creatinine is a waste product removed from the blood by healthy kidneys. A creatinine blood test greater than 1.2 for women is a sign of kidney disease. Another test that looks for blood urea nitrogen (BUN) is also important; when the BUN "rises," so to speak, it's a sign of kidney disease. Other more sensitive tests that detect the level of kidney function include creatinine clearance, glomerular filtration rate (GFR), and urine albumin.

Treating Kidney Disease

If you have high blood pressure, getting it under control through diet, exercise, or blood pressure–lowering strategies will help to save your kidneys. In general, slowing the progression of kidney disease can be done by the following:

✦ Controlling high blood pressure (see Chapter 2).

✦ Controlling blood sugar levels (see Chapter 1).

✦ Adopting a kidney-smart diet (see "What to Eat" in this chapter).

✦ Treating urinary tract infections (see Chapter 7).

✦ Exercise and weight loss (see "How to Move" in Chapters 2 and 3).

From Kidney Disease to Kidney Failure

Kidney failure is also known as chronic renal insufficiency (CRI); this term means that your kidneys are functioning at 50 percent or less than normal capacity. By this point, your kidneys are working with "half the staff" and are not able to remove bodily wastes as efficiently as a healthy kidney. Again, you may not notice symptoms of kidney failure at all; the disease progresses slowly and, as the kidneys continue to fail and more waste products build up, you'll begin to feel sick. Because your kidneys stop making enough of the crucial hormone erythropoietin (EPO), you can suffer from low iron levels or anemia as well as weakness. When the kidneys are functioning at less than 10 percent of their capacity, you'll need to consider dialysis or even a kidney transplant. By this point, you've progressed to end-stage renal disease.

WHAT TO EAT

To prolong the life of your kidneys when you experience signs of kidney disease or are in the early stages (and perhaps have been alerted through blood test results), you can adjust your diet to cut down on the work your kidneys normally do as well as meet nutritional needs, such as increasing iron intake, which may be lower due to anemia. Diet can even control the buildup of food wastes and reduce fatigue, nausea, itching, and a bad taste in the mouth that can occur when toxins build up in the body. Of course, diet will also help to control high blood sugar. When you think about a kidney-smart diet, remember "3PS," a term I've coined to remember protein, potassium, phosphorus, and sodium. The diet involves *cutting down on 3PS*. A dietitian or nutritionist can help you make the cuts necessary to save your kidneys, but keep you as healthy as possible.

Protein

Protein is a good thing normally; it builds, repairs, and maintains your body tissues, and it also helps you fight infections or heal wounds. But as protein breaks down in the body, it forms urea, which is a waste product. The kidney normally flushes out urea. When it can't, urea builds up in the blood, so cutting down on protein is necessary. You need to eat enough for health, however. Meat, fish, poultry, eggs, tofu, and dairy products are high in protein.

Potassium

Your nerves and muscles normally rely on the mineral potassium to work well. But without the filtering process of your kidneys, too much can build up in your blood, which can affect your heart. Normally your kidneys get rid of potassium excess, so most of us never think about it. But when your kidneys aren't functioning well, we can cut down on potassium-rich foods, such as potatoes, squash, bananas, oranges, tomatoes, dried peas, and beans.

Phosphorus (phosphate)

Your bones normally rely on the mineral phosphorus to stay healthy and strong. When phosphorus levels rise, usually the kidneys just filter out excess phosphorus and we feel fine. But when the kidneys aren't working well, phosphorus levels rise until we get itchy skin or painful joints. Limiting foods with phosphorus will help reduce toxic levels of this mineral. These foods include anything with protein, such as seeds, nuts, dried peas, beans, and processed bran cereals. You'll need some phosphorus-containing foods for health. When you ingest them, you can also take a phosphate binder, a medication that binds with the phosphorus in your intestine so it can pass in your stool. Ask your doctor about prescribing a binder.

Sodium

As discussed in the high blood pressure section in an earlier chapter, sodium affects your body fluids and blood pressure. Reducing sodium means cutting down on salt and packaged or canned products with sodium (canned soups are notorious). Start reading labels and stop salting your foods. Avoid foods with a high sodium content. Processed foods, such as deli meats, fast foods, salty snacks, and anything with salty seasonings, are high in sodium. There are many herbs you can use instead; lemon and vinegar are terrific substitutes, too.

Fluids

Kidneys produce urine, which eliminates many of our wastes. When kidneys are not functioning well, not as much urine is produced, and this can cause fluid retention—swelling in hands, legs, feet, and so on. Limiting your fluid intake may help, but it isn't necessary in all cases. Fluids include water, soup, juice, milk, popsicles, and gelatin; you and your doctor should discuss how to limit your fluid intake.

Vitamins and Minerals

People with kidney disease are frequently deficient in B_6. Vitamin B_6 is also available as a supplement. (See Appendix A for food sources.)

FLOWER POWER

The following herbs are good for the kidneys and bladder:

Couch grass.   Meadowsweet.

Cranberry.   Uva Ursi.

The following essential oils are good for the kidneys (see methods of use on p. 51):

Clary sage.

Generaium.

Grapefruit.

Juniper (not recommended if you are in kidney failure).

Lemongrass.

How to Move

The best exercises for kidney health are hands-on healing in the form of massage or acupuncture, which can stimulate the qi or life force energy to the kidneys. (See Chapter 3 for more information on qi gong and acupuncture.)

CHAPTER SEVEN

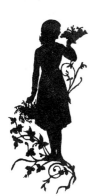

Staying Sexy Naturally

Diabetes can wreak havoc on your sex life, which is imperative for quality of life and self-esteem when women are managing diabetes. Thirty percent of women with diabetes suffer from sexual dysfunction due to either vaginal or bladder problems related to diabetes complications. This chapter discusses the range of diabetes-related problems below the belt and offers natural solutions through diet, exercises, and herbal approaches.

Vagina Problems

Nerve damage can affect arousal for women. Special nerve fibers and blood vessels connect to the clitoris, vaginal wall, and vulva, which are necessary for achieving orgasm and lubrication. If you have sustained nerve damage, you may notice a loss of sensation in your genital area, which can be a frustrating experience. Phytoestrogens (see "Flower Power" later in this chapter), natural progesterone therapy (see page 152), and lubricants may help, as well as trying different positions to increase arousal.

Vaginal dryness has a domino effect: The dryness itself can increase your vulnerability to yeast infections. Dry vaginas can be torn during intercourse, and the resultant wounds can become vulnerable to yeast infection. High blood sugar levels also increase the amount of sugar in the vaginal walls, which can also cause yeast infections.

Note: Antibiotics prescribed to women for the purposes of clearing up a bladder infection can predispose them to yeast infections, too, a classic side effect that all women can experience when they take antibiotics for any reason.

Yeast Infections

Yeast infections are caused by a yeast known as *candida albicans,* a one-cell fungus that belongs to the plant kingdom. Under normal circumstances, candida is always in your vagina, mouth, and digestive tract. It is "friendly" fungus. For a variety of reasons, candida will overgrow and reproduce too much of itself, changing from a harmless one-cell fungus into long branches of yeast cells called mycelia. This is known as *candidiasis.*

Generally, any changes to your vagina's normal acidic environment can make you vulnerable to candidiasis. The list of factors that affect your vaginal environment is quite long. High blood sugar levels increase the amount of sugar stored in the vaginal cell walls, and yeast *loves* sugar. In fact, women who suffer from chronic yeast infections are encouraged to be screened for diabetes because they are so common in women with diabetes.

Anything that interferes with the immune system will make yeast thrive, too. Antibiotics, for example, not only kill the harmful bacteria, but often the friendly bacteria that are always in the vagina and that are necessary to fend off infection.

Severe itching and a curdlike or cottage-cheesy discharge are classic symptoms of candidiasis. The discharge, interestingly, may also smell like baking bread, fermenting yeast, or even brewing beer. So if the discharge is foul-smelling or fishy, you can rule out yeast. The discharge may also be thinner and mucus-like, but it is always white. Other symptoms are swelling, redness, and irritation of the outer and inner vaginal lips, painful sex, and painful urination due to an irritation of the urethra.

When yeast is in the throat, it is called *thrush* and usually occurs in immune-suppressed women (they may possibly be HIV-positive or undergoing cancer treatments). Thrush is unsettling because the mouth and throat are coated with a milky-white goop. Yeast infections can be controlled through diet and herbal supplements (see "What to Eat" and "Flower Power" later in this chapter).

Bladder Problems

Sexual dysfunction in women is also related to nerve damage to the bladder. When the bladder is not emptied sufficiently, it leads to bacterial bladder infections or urinary tract infections, which makes sex uncomfortable. Nerves that control the bladder can be affected, causing you to lose your sense of bladder urge and your ability to force a bladder contraction (that is, to urinate). Ultimately this can lead to incontinence, as urine will start to leak out. Learning to go to the bathroom on a schedule (every four hours or so), instead of waiting for the urge, is one solution. (There are several bladder control/strengthening exercises listed under "How to Move.")

Regardless of diabetes, roughly 75 percent of women will experience one or more incidents of urinary incontinence after menopause. This may result in "stress incontinence" (leakage when laughing, sneezing, coughing, running, picking up something, and other normal activities that put stress on the bladder). It may also be experienced as "urge incontinence" (leakage as soon as the urge comes on, except that there is no time to get to the toilet). Damaged or weakened pelvic-floor muscles, which many women damage during childbirth, are the causes. Other aggravating factors include alcohol use, urinary tract infections, fibroids, and chronic constipation.

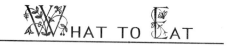

What to Eat

To Prevent/Control Yeast Infections

Plain yogurt, an antifungal, is the best way to fend off yeast. Simply eat a small container of any kind of yogurt daily; as long as it has active bacterial culture, any brand is fine. Alternatively, you can take *lactobacillus acidophilus*, which is generally available in capsule form at any drug store. If you find that you have thrush, citrus seed extract and tea-tree oil can be used in a gargle.

Following an "anti-yeast" diet may also be helpful. Certain foods interfere with the vagina's acidity, something you need to prevent yeast. The diet entails avoiding the following: sugar, honey, maple syrup, molasses, and any foods that contain them; alcoholic beverages; vinegars and foods containing vinegar, such as pickled foods, salad dressings, mustard, ketchup, and mayonnaise; moldy nuts, such as peanuts, pistachios, and cashews; soy sauce, miso, and other fermented products; dairy food with the exception of butter, buttermilk, and yogurt; coffee, black tea, and sweetened soda pop; dried fruits; and processed foods.

Try to incorporate more of the following foods to compensate: whole grains, such as rice, millet, barley, and buckwheat; breads, crackers, and muffins that are yeast-free and preferably wheat-free; raw or cooked fresh vegetables; fish, chicken, and lean meats (organically fed and hormone- and antibiotic-free); nuts and seeds that are not moldy; and fruit in moderation (limiting sweeter fruits).

For Vaginal Dryness and Irritation (or Vaginitis)

Avoid the following, as they aggravate vaginal dryness:

✦ Coffee.

✦ Alcohol.

✦ White sugar.

✦ Severe stress (see Chapter 1).

✦ Steroid/cortisone drugs. (Note: Vaginal anti-itch creams contain cortisol and should be used as a last resort; cortisone contributes to osteoporosis.)

Natural "household" vaginal lubricants—in your kitchen

✦ Coconut oil.

✦ Raw egg white.

✦ Honey.

✦ Olive oil.

✦ Vegetable oil.

✦ Vitamin E oil.

✦ Each day, ingest some omega-3 fatty acids, such as flax-seed oils.

For Severe Itching

✦ Drink only water for beverages.

✦ Drink a special "rice broth," which works as an internal moisturizer. Boil a small handful of rice in 16 oz/500 ml or more of water to make a thin broth.

Vitamins and Minerals

Vitamin B_{12} supplements help with vaginal lubrication. (See Appendix A for food sources.)

For Bladder Control

Avoid the following bladder irritants: (Also note that smoking increases your risk of developing stress incontinence by 350 percent.)

- ✦ Caffeine.
- ✦ Alcohol.
- ✦ White sugar.
- ✦ Citrus.
- ✦ Tomatoes.
- ✦ Cayenne.
- ✦ Hot peppers.
- ✦ Iced drinks.
- ✦ Carbonated drinks.
- ✦ Pineapple.

Note: Many common drugs trigger incontinence, among them diuretics, antidepressants, beta-blockers, blood pressure–lowering drugs, sleeping pills, and tranquilizers.

FLOWER POWER

The following help with lubrication and to relieve itching:

- ✦ Aloe vera gel (bottled or fresh).

- ✦ Acidophilus capsules inserted vaginally help prevent yeast infections and create copious amounts of lubrication. Insert one or two between two and four hours before love-making.

- ✦ Comfrey root sitz bath. Brew two quarts/liters of the infusion, rewarm, strain, and soak in a "sitz" for five to 10 minutes several times a week.

✦ Before making love, chew on a piece of Dang Gui root to increase vaginal lubrication.

✦ Use chickweed tincture, 25 to 40 drops in water, several times a day for two to four weeks.

✦ Twenty-five drops motherwort tincture or one to three teaspoons of safflower or flax seed oil can help to increase vaginal lubrication and thicken vaginal walls.

✦ Comfrey ointment. Rub in morning and night and use as a lubricant. The vulva will be noticeably plumper and moister within three weeks.

✦ Use slippery elm as a soothing vaginal gel. Slowly heat two tablespoons slippery elm bark in a cup of water, stirring until thick. Cool before spreading over and inside the vulva and vagina. The gel lubricates, heals, and nourishes.

✦ Mix essential oil of *Salvia sclarea* with olive oil and apply it to dry vaginal tissues that have lost their elasticity.

To Relieve *Severe* Vaginal Itching and Burning

✦ Belladonna.

✦ Cantharis.

✦ Sulfur.

✦ Natrum mur.

✦ Motherwort tincture. Ten to 20 drops several times a day.

✦ Plantian oil or ointment.

✦ Brew a quart/liter of nettle infusion several times a week. Either sit in it through a sitz bath or drink it.

+ Calendula cream applied morning and evening.

+ Take an oat or honey bath. (You can put honey on a pad and wear it, as it draws in moisture.)

+ Comfrey root or chamomile blossom compress. Infuse the comfrey and soak a towel in it, or make some chamomile tea and use the teabag. Apply either.

To Strengthen Bladder

+ Pulsatilla.

+ Zincum.

+ Boil dried teasel (*Dipsacus sylvestris*) roots with a tablespoon to a cup of water for 10 to 15 minutes and then drink daily.

+ Replace your coffee with cranberry juice.

+ Antispasmodic herbs such as black cohosh, ginger, catnip, and cornsilk may urge incontinence.

+ Yarrow (*Achillea milefolium*) will help heal bladder infections, incontinence, and heavy periods but may aggravate hot flashes. Recommended as a tea or infusion of the dried flowers as desired, or as a tincture of the fresh flowering tops, five to 10 drops, two to three times daily.

Natural Progesterone

Natural progesterone helps to restore vaginal tone, lubrication, and bladder control. In our bodies, progesterone helps to regulate blood sugar levels, something that can be counterbalanced when we have too much estrogen in our bodies. Natural progesterone therapy is an alternative for relieving many women's health problems, including PMS, menopause symptoms, and the estrogen-loss ailments associated with menopause.

Natural progesterone therapy is not available everywhere. You can't just walk into a healthfood store and buy natural progesterone. It needs to be prescribed by a doctor (although the doctor need not be an M.D.; several naturopathic doctors are prescribing them, too). A pharmacist has to prepare a doctor's prescription for natural progesterone from scratch. This is known as a compounding pharmacist. Not all pharmacies are "compounding pharmacies," so ask your doctor or current pharmacist about where to go to get a prescription prepared. You can also call the International Academy of Coumpounding Pharmacists (IACP) or the Professional Compunding Centers of America, Inc. (PCCA) for the nearest compounding pharmacist in your area. Several Canadian compounding pharmacists are members of either or both organizations. You can reach the PCCA at (800) 331-2498 or at *www.pccarx.com.*

What you can get over the counter in some healthfood stores and natural pharmacies are creams containing botanical progesterone, which is progesterone that comes from plants such as wild yam. This is not harmful, but it will not be as pure as the progesterone your doctor prescribes, which often comes from soy and wild yam, too, but is a very *pure* extraction. The term natural does not mean "human"; it means that it is not synthetic. Natural progesterone is recognized by our progesterone receptors as if it were progesterone we made in our bodies.

Creams

Progesterone works very well in cream form. There are few kinds:

✦ Creams that contain only progesterone in a carrier such as aloe vera or vitamin E.

+ Creams that contain progesterone and other essential oils or herbs.

+ Creams that contain progesterone and phyoestrogens (plant estrogens).

+ Creams that contain progesterone and three kinds of natural estrogen.

Creams that contain estrogen are not for you; they're for menopausal women who are using natural hormone therapy to relieve estrogen loss and other menopausal discomforts.

Natural progesterone can also be found in an oil form (taken under the tongue); tablets, capsules, vaginal suppositories, a vaginal gel, and an injectable form.

Other Supplements

✧ Polycarbophil, the active ingredient in many over-the-counter vaginal creams, pulls water into vaginal cells, helping to restore and maintain healthy lubrication. It also reduces vaginal infections by making the vagina more alkaline.

✧ Estrogens creams are available everywhere. The only problem is that even when applied vaginally, they are absorbed by the blood and will carry many of the same risks as taking oral estrogens. So if you do not want estrogen side effects, this may not be the best route. You can also purchase estrogen and testosterone creams.

How to Move

In this situation, moving your pelvic muscles can help to improve vaginal and bladder tone.

Exercises to Improve Pelvic Muscles

1. Try to bring yourself to an orgasm alone or with a partner.

2. Pelvic-Floor Exercises:

   ◆ Breathe out and push down as though you were trying to push something out of your vagina. Hold for three seconds, then inhale and relax. Do 25 to 50 reps.

   ◆ To tone vaginal muscles and increase lubrication, tighten the inner muscles of the vagina around a finger or small, smooth marble and hold for 10 to 13 seconds; pulse (contract and relax) your vaginal muscles rapidly (10 to 30 times) as you breathe out. Repeat 10 to 25 times.

   ◆ To tone vagina and bladder: sit in a bathtub with water up to your hips. See if you can suck water into your vagina and expel it. Suck in as you breathe in; push out as you breathe out. Do 25 to 50 times.

Exercises to Improve Bladder Control or Incontinence

1. Pelvic-floor exercises (see the previous section).

2. While-you-pee exercises:

   ◆ Kegel Exercises: Isolate the tiny muscles that start and stop your urinary stream. (In other words, the next time you pee, stop the flow.) Hold as long as you can (work up to at least 10 seconds) before letting go and peeing again. Practice this every time you urinate. (You can also do this when you're not urinating to strengthen the muscle.)

- ◆ Pulse your urine flow by pushing out very strongly, then slackening it off until it's just a dribble, then push out again, and so on. Repeat as many times as possible every time you urinate.

- ◆ Empty the bladder completely every time by pressing down behind your pubic bone with fingertips or the flat of your palm.

- ◆ Scheduled toileting: go on a regular schedule, say, every 60 to 90 minutes. After three to four consecutive dry days, increase the interval by 15 to 30 minutes, and keep increasing until you're at every four hours.

3. Other exercises:

- ◆ Push hard on the very top of the head to relieve urge incontinence on the spot.

- ◆ Set out two shallow basins: one with very hot water, the other with cold. Start by relaxing for three minutes in the hot one. Then lower yourself up and down, in and out of the icy water for one minute. Repeat three to four times; do this several times a week.

Tips to Avoid Yeast Infections

✧ *Don't wear tight clothing around your vagina.* Tight pants, panties, and nylon pantyhose prevent your vagina from breathing and make it warmer and moister for yeast. Wear looser pants that allow your vagina to breathe, switch to knee highs or old-fashioned stockings, or wear pantyhose only for special occasions. Go "bottomless" to bed to let air into your vagina.

✧ *Wear only 100-percent cotton clothing and/or natural fibers around your vagina.* Synthetic underwear and polyester pants are not good ideas. All cotton underwear, denim, wool, or rayon pants that are loose-fitting are fine.

✧ *Avoid vaginal deodorants or sprays.* These products are unnecessary and disturb the vagina's natural environment, which is fully designed to "self-clean."

✧ *Don't douche unless it's for purely medicinal purposes.* Douching can push harmful bacteria up higher into the vagina, disturb the vagina's natural ecosystem, or interfere with a pregnancy.

✧ *Watch your toilet habits.* Always wipe from front to back with toilet paper. When you do it the other way around, you can introduce fecal material and germs into your vagina. After a looser bowel movement, wet the toilet paper and clean your rectal area thoroughly so that fecal material doesn't stay on your underwear and wind up in your vagina. If you are in a less hygienic bathroom that doesn't have running water near the toilet, spit on your toilet paper and clean the rectal area. (It's better than nothing.)

✧ *Don't insert anything into a dry vagina.* Whether it's a penis or a tampon, make sure your vagina is well lubricated before insertion.

✧ Avoid wearing tampons.

✧ *Avoid long car trips on vinyl seats.* New research indicates that vinyl seats increase a woman's risk of developing a yeast infection because the vinyl traps moisture and does not allow the crotch area to breathe.

CHAPTER EIGHT

Foot Notes

Foot complications related to diabetes were dramatized in the mid-1980s film *Nothing in Common*, in which Jackie Gleason plays the ne'er-do-well diabetic father, and Tom Hanks plays the son who cannot accept him. In a heartbreaking scene, Tom Hanks is shocked to discover how ill his father really is when he finally sees his feet. They are swollen, purple, and badly infected. Ultimately, the story ends with the father and son coming to terms as Gleason must undergo surgical amputation.

I share this example with you because many of us are used to ignoring and abusing our feet. We wear uncomfortable shoes, we pick at our calluses and blisters, we don't wear socks with our shoes, and so on. You can't do this any more. Your feet are the targets of both macrovascular (large blood vessel) complications and microvascular (small blood vessel) complications. In the first case, peripheral vascular disease affects blood circulation to your feet. In the second place, the nerve cells to your feet, which control sensation, can be altered through microvascular complications. Nerve damage can also affect your feet's muscles and tendons, causing weakness and changes to your foot's shape.

What Can Happen to Your Feet

The combination of poor circulation and numbness in your feet means that you can sustain an injury to your feet and not know it. For example, you might step on a piece of glass or badly stub your toe and not realize it. If an open wound becomes infected and you have poor circulation, the wound will not heal properly, and infection could spread to the bone or gangrene could develop. (In this situation, amputation may be the only treatment.) Or, without sensation or proper circulation in them, your feet could be far more vulnerable to frostbite or exposure than they would be otherwise. Diabetes can also cause your feet to thicken as a result of poor circulation. In this case the skin on the foot becomes very thin and blood vessels are visible through the skin, which has a shiny appearance and looks red. Thinner skin can be more easily pierced and infected.

As if this weren't enough for your feet, they can also be damaged from bone loss: osteoporosis of the feet! Diabetes can cause your body to take more calcium from bones. Because there are 26 bones in your foot alone, bone loss in the foot can weaken it, and it can break more easily or become deformed with bigger arches and a claw-like toe. All of this can cause calluses that can get infected, leading to gangrene and amputation, too.

Diabetes accounts for approximately half of all non-emergency amputations, but all experts agree that doing a foot self-exam every day (see "The Foot Self-Exam," following) can prevent most foot complications from becoming severe. Those most at risk for foot problems are people who smoke (smoking aggravates *all* diabetic complications) or who are overweight (overweight people with diabetes have a 5- to 15-percent risk of undergoing amputation during their lifetime). Roughly 80 percent of diabetes-related amputations could have been prevented with proper foot care.

Signs of Foot Problems

The most common symptoms of foot complications are burning, tingling, or pain in your feet or legs. These are all signs of nerve damage. Numbness is another symptom that could mean nerve damage or circulation problems. If you do experience pain from nerve damage, it usually gets worse with time (as new nerves and blood vessels grow), and many people find that it's worse at night. Bed linens can actually increase discomfort. Some people notice foot symptoms only after exercising or a short walk, but many people don't notice immediate symptoms until they've lost feeling in their feet.

Other symptoms people notice are frequent infections (caused by blood-vessel damage), hair loss on the toes or lower legs, or shiny skin on the lower legs and feet. Foot deformity or open wounds on the feet are also signs.

When You Knock Your Socks Off

When you take off your socks at the end of the day, get in the habit of doing a foot self-exam. This is the only way you can do damage control on your feet. You're looking for signs of infection or potential infection triggers. If you can avoid infection at all costs, you will be able to keep your feet. Look for the following signs:

- ✦ Reddened, discolored, or swollen areas (blue, bright red, or white areas mean that circulation is cut off).
- ✦ Pus.
- ✦ Temperature changes in the feet or "hot spots."
- ✦ Corns, calluses, and warts. (Potential infections could be hiding under calluses. Do not remove these yourself; see a podiatrist.)
- ✦ Toenails that are too long. (Your toenail could cut you if it's too long.)

✦ Redness where your shoes or socks are rubbing due to a poor fit. (When your sock is scrunched inside your shoe, the folds could actually rub against the skin and cause a blister.)

✦ Toenail fungus (under the nail).

✦ Fungus between the toes (athlete's foot, common if you've been walking around barefoot in a public place).

✦ Breaks in the skin (especially between your toes), or cracks, such as in calluses on the heels. (These open the door for bacteria.)

If you find an infection, wash your feet carefully with soap and water; *don't use alcohol*. Then see your doctor or a podiatrist (a foot specialist) as soon as possible. If your foot is irritated but not yet infected (redness, for example, from poor-fitting shoes but no blister yet), simply avoid the irritant—the shoes—and it should clear up. If not, see your doctor. If you're overweight and have trouble inspecting your feet, get somebody else to check them for the signs previously listed. In addition to doing a self-exam, see your doctor to have the circulation and reflexes in your feet checked four times a year.

The Foot Self-Exam (FSE)

Ever heard of a breast self-exam? Well, this is a foot self-exam you can do that I've compiled from different sources. Do this each day and you can prevent serious foot complications:

✦ Look for redness. Redness is a sign of irritation or pending breaks in the skin.

✦ Look for breaks in the skin, which include blisters or cracks, especially between the toes. They can become infected.

✦ Look for calluses, which could turn into sores or blisters.

+ Look for changes in foot shape, such as deformity.

+ Look for signs of swelling, which could also mean fluid retention related to kidney disease (see Chapter 7).

+ Wash your feet and lower legs every day in lukewarm water with mild soap. Dry them really well, especially between the toes.

+ Baby your feet. When the skin seems too moist, use baby powder or a foot powder your doctor or pharmacist recommends (especially between the toes). When your feet are too dry, moisturize them with a lotion recommended by your doctor or pharmacist. The reason is simple: Breaks in the skin happen if feet are too moist (such as between the toes) or too dry (such as cracking). Use a foot-buffing pad on your calluses after bathing.

When You Have an Open Wound

Open wounds on the feet are also called "foot ulcers" and affect millions of people with diabetes; about 20 percent of diabetes-related foot ulcers don't heal, leading to amputation to prevent gangrene. Any tear in the skin can lead to an open wound that becomes infected. Blisters, cracks in the feet from dryness, and stepping on something sharp are the most common causes of open wounds.

Healing Open Wounds

The first order of business is to remove the source of irritation that caused the sore, such as bad shoes or poor hygiene (see "How to Move" later in this chapter). Dressing the wound well (cleaning it, using proper bandages, and so on) and using natural substances with antibiotic properties may also help.

(This book is only reporting on drug-free remedies, but over-the-counter antibiotics may be necessary.) Keeping pressure off the feet can also help to heal them. Often healing a foot ulcer requires home care; you may need to have a nurse or home healthcare worker come into your home and dress your wounds. When wounds are open and not healing well, a very unpleasant odor can develop. Waiting for your daily dressing while you heal your foot sore can be pretty isolating and depressing for many people. One experience with this is often enough for you to take prevention steps seriously.

What to Eat

First and foremost, keeping your blood sugar under control is the key to avoiding foot problems (review Chapter 1). Next, follow a heart-smart diet (outlined in Chapter 2); this will improve circulation.

Increase Your Calcium Intake

Calcium will help keep the bones in your feet strong; if you're past menopause, it can also help to prevent osteoporosis. Four glasses of milk are equal to about 1,200 mg of calcium. When you're trying to increase calcium in your diet, you also need to avoid substances that cause you to use up or "pee out" calcium, such as alcohol or coffee.

Maximizing Calcium Absorption

Calcium is best absorbed in an acidic environment. To increase acidity:

✦ Add two tablespoons/30 ml of apple cider vinegar and two tablespoons raw honey or blackstrap molasses to a cup/250 ml water; drink with or after your meal.

+ Drink lemon juice in water with or after your meal.

+ Use calcium-rich herbal vinegars in your salad dressing.

Calcium greens

+ Broccoli, kale, turnip greens, or mustard greens contains about 200 mg calcium. One cup cooked collards, wild onions, lamb's quarter, or amaranth greens have about 400 mg calcium.

+ The following greens are not high calcium sources, but high iron sources: spinach, swiss chard (silver beet), beet greens, and wood sorrel.

High-Calcium Sources

Some of these you probably know about; many of these you don't.

+ Tahini.

+ Soy or tofu (not all tofu contains calcium; check labels).

+ Oats/oatmeal.

+ Seaweed.

+ Sardines.

+ Yogurt.

+ Nettles.

+ Dandelion leaves.

+ Dried fruit (65 mg of calcium can be found in three small figs, a handful of raisins, four dates, or eight prunes).

+ Corn tortillas. (Because these are made with lime, these are high in calcium.)

Calcium Supplements

If you can't get enough calcium in your diet, there are always supplements. Calcium supplements are more effective in divided doses. Two doses of 250 mg, taken morning and night, actually provide more usable calcium than a 1,000 mg tablet. New research also shows that the amount of calcium absorbed from calcium citrate supplements is consistently higher than the amount absorbed from calcium carbonate supplements. Popular supplements include:

✦ Calcium-fortified orange juice. This is easier to digest and absorb than other supplements.

✦ Calcium citrate in tablet form (crushed tablets are better absorbed).

✦ Calcium gluconate, calcium lactate, and calcium carbonate (if chewable). You can take 1,500 mg daily of one of these.

FLOWER POWER

You can add the following calcium-rich herbs to your diet:

✦ Nettle.

✦ Sage.

✦ Chickweed.

✦ Red clover.

✦ Comfrey leaf.

✦ Raspberry leaf.

✦ Oatstraw.

Note: A big mug of infusion using any of these herbs is equal to 250 to 300 mg calcium. Add a big pinch of horsetail and increase the calcium by 10 percent.

The Uni-Tea Company makes a calcium-rich tea called FemininiTea that contains raspberry leaves, nettles, ginger, licorice, chamomile, sarsaparilla, rosemary, rose petals, yellow dock, uva ursi, dong quai, peony, lavender, and angelica. You can find this product in some health food or natural food stores.

Healing wounds

Review Chapter 3 for herbs that promote wound-healing.

Essential Oils

For calluses, you can massage chamomile, fennel, lavender, or lemon onto the foot. For corns, lemon oil is recommended. To control foot odor, baking powder with sage, mixed first in a baggie and then sprinkled in shoes, is helpful.

How to Move

By following these steps, you can prevent diabetes foot complications:

✦ Walk a little bit every day; this is a good way to improve blood flow and get a little exercise!

✦ Don't walk around barefoot; wear proper-fitting, clean, cotton socks with your shoes daily, and get in the habit of wearing slippers around the house and shoes at the beach. If you're swimming, wear some sort of shoe (plastic "jellies" or canvas running shoes). This doesn't mean you have to look like the geek who wears white sports socks with Greek sandals; there are lots of options. If it's cold out, wear woolen socks.

✦ Before you put on your shoes, shake them out in case something such as your (grand)child's Lego piece, a piece of dry cat food, or a pebble is in there.

✦ Trim your toenails straight across to avoid ingrown nails. Don't pick off your nails. Use only a nail clipper, and be sure not to cut into the corners of the nails. Use a nail file or emery board to smooth or round rough edges.

✦ No more "bathroom surgery" on your feet, which may include puncturing blisters with needles or tweezers, shaving your calluses, and the hundreds of crazy things people do to their feet (but never disclose to their spouses).

✦ When you're sitting down, feet should be flat on the floor. Sitting cross-legged or in crossed-legged variations can cut off your circulation (and frequently does, even in people without diabetes).

✦ Wear comfortable, proper-fitting footwear. See the box on page 169 for tips about shoe shopping.

✦ Avoid heat. Extreme heat, such as heating pads, very hot water, and even hot sun, can cause swelling or burn your feet.

✦ Don't wear clothing that restricts blood flow to your legs and feet, including girdles, garters, tight pantyhose, or socks that cut off the circulation.

✦ If you're overweight, lose some weight; it puts less pressure on your feet.

How to Shoe Shop for Health

To save your feet, you may not be able to save on your next pair of shoes. These are new shoe-shopping rules:

- ✧ Shoe shop at the time of day when your feet are most swollen (such as the afternoon). That way, you'll purchase a shoe that fits you in "bad times" as well as good times.
- ✧ Don't even think about high heels or any type of shoe that is not comfortable or that doesn't fit properly. Say goodbye to thongs. That strip between your toe can cause too much irritation.
- ✧ Buy leather; avoid shoes with the terms "man-made upper" or "man-made materials" on the label; this means that the shoes are made of synthetic materials and your foot will not breathe. Cotton or canvas shoes are fine as long as the insole is cotton, too. Man-made materials on the very bottom of the shoe are fine as long as the upper—the part of the shoe that touches your foot—is leather, cotton, canvas, or something breathable.
- ✧ Remember that leather does, indeed, stretch. When that happens, the shoe can become loose and cause blisters. On the other hand, if the shoe is too tight and the salesperson tells you the shoe will stretch, forget it. The shoe will destroy you in the first few hours of wear, which sort of "defeets" the purpose.
- ✧ If you lose all sensation and cannot feel whether the shoe is fitting, make sure you have a shoe salesperson fit you.
- ✧ Avoid shoes that have been on display. A variety of people try these shoes on; you never know what bacteria and fungi these shoes harbor.

Getting an Artificial Limb

Artificial limbs are also called prosthetic limbs or simply a prosthesis. In the United States, some of the costs for the prosthesis may be covered by your health insurance plan. You can also look into non-profit agencies for help.

Doctors do not have prosthetic limbs you can purchase. You have to go to a special artisan of sorts, known as an orthotist or prosthetist, a person who is trained in making artificial limbs and understands amputees' needs. The orthotist or prosthetist must have a doctor's prescription before he or she makes the limb.

Some prosthetic companies have catalogs, allowing you to order direct and sometimes bypassing the prescription, but it's best to be fitted for a limb in person and to work directly with a prosthetist. Ordering from the Internet or a catalog is akin to ordering a breast implant from a catalog. You should be fitted. Amputees recommend shopping around for an orthotist or prosthetist; the limb prices vary wildly from manufacturer to manufacturer and prosthetist to prosthetist.

Most prosthetists are willing to work with you and answer the many questions you may have about how the limb is made, durability, ranges of motions, and so on.

17 Questions to Ask
When Shopping for Artificial Limbs

1. What is the alignment of the limb? This refers to the position of prosthetic socket in relation to foot and knee.

2. Is the equipment assistive or adaptive? This refers to devices that assist in performance or mobility, including ramps and bars, changes in furniture heights, environmental control units, and specially designed devices.

3. Will you prepare a check socket, or test socket? This is a trial socket, which is often transparent, made to evaluate comfort and fit prior to the final prosthesis design.

4. What is a control cable? This is a steel cable used to move and lock mechanical joints and to operate body-powered prostheses.

5. What material will you use for the cosmetic cover? This refers to the material from which the surface of the limb is made, giving it a more natural appearance. Materials used could be plastic, foam, rubber laminate, or stocking. An endoskeletal limb is one in which the prosthesis consists of a lightweight plastic or metal tube encased in a foam cover. An exoskeletal limb is a prosthesis made of plastic over wood or rigid foam.

6. Will it be made with energy-storing feet? This refers to prosthetic feet with plastic springs or carbon fibers designed to help move the prosthesis forward.

7. Will it be designed with knee components? This refers to devices designed to create a safe, smooth walking pattern.

8. Will it have a single axis? This refers to a free-swinging knee with a small amount of friction.

17 Questions to Ask
When Shopping for Artificial Limbs (cont.)

9. Will it have stance control? This refers to a friction device with an adjustable brake mechanism to add stability.

10. Will this limb be polycentric? This refers to a multiple-axis joint, which is particularly useful with a very long residual limb.

11. Will it have manual locking? This refers to a device that locks the knee in complete extension to prevent buckling and falls.

12. Will it have pneumatic or hydraulic controls? This provides controlled changes in the speed of walking.

13. Will it be a myoelectric prosthesis? This means it has electrodes mounted within the socket to receive signals from muscle contraction to control a motor in the terminal device, wrist rotator, or elbow.

14. Will it have nudge control? This is a mechanical switch that operates one or more joints of the prosthesis.

15. Will I see a preparatory prosthesis before the definitive prosthesis? *Definitive* means the final product, which meets accepted clinical standards for comfort, fit, alignment, function, appearance, and durability. A *preparatory* prosthesis refers to a short-term prosthesis, generally without cosmetic finishing, that is provided in the early phase of fitting to expedite prosthetic wear and use; it also aids in the evaluation of amputee adjustment and component selection.

17 Questions to Ask
When Shopping for Artificial Limbs (cont.)

16. How is the socket constructed? This refers to a portion of the prosthesis that fits around the residual limb or stump and to which prosthetic components are attached. A "hard socket" is a prosthetic socket made of rigid materials; a "soft socket" refers to the inner socket liner of foam, rubber, leather, or other material for cushioning the residual limb.

17. What materials will be designed to protect my residual limb (or "stump")? Ask about things such as a stockinette (a tubular open-ended cotton or nylon material); a stump sock (a wool or cotton sock worn over a residual limb to provide a cushion between the skin and socket interface); and a stump shrinker (an elastic wrap or compression sock worn on a residual limb to reduce swelling and shape the limb).

Source: Questions compiled from material retrieved from The Amputee Web Site, *www.amputee-online.ca,* July 2001.

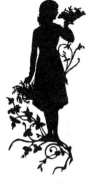

Where to Find Your Vitamins and Minerals

VITAMIN/MINERAL	**Vitamin A/Beta Carotene.**
FOUND IN	Liver, fish oils, egg yolks, whole milk, butter; Beta Carotene-leafy greens, yellow and orange vegetables and fruits.
HERBAL SOURCES OF	Peppermint, yellow dock, uva ursi, parsley, alfalfa, raspberry leaves, nettles, dandelion greens, kelp, green onions, violet leaves, cayenne, paprika, sage, chickweed, lamb's quarters, horsetail, black cohosh, rose hips.
DEPLETED BY	Coffee, alcohol, cortisone, mineral oil, fluorescent lights, liver "cleansing," excessive intake of iron, lack of protein.

VITAMIN/MINERAL	**Vitamin B$_6$.**
FOUND IN	Meats, poultry, fish, nuts, liver, bananas, avocados, grapes, pears, egg yolk, whole grains, legumes.
HERBAL SOURCES OF	Wheat germ, seeds, soybeans.
DEPLETED BY	Coffee, alcohol, tobacco, sugar, raw oysters, birth control pills.

VITAMIN/MINERAL	**Vitamin B$_{12}$.**
FOUND IN	Meats, dairy products, eggs, liver, fish.
HERBAL SOURCES OF	Wheat germ, seeds, soybeans, miso.
DEPLETED BY	Coffee, alcohol, tobacco, sugar, raw oysters, birth control pills.

VITAMIN/MINERAL	**Vitamin C.**
FOUND IN	Citrus fruits, broccoli, green pepper, strawberries, cabbage, tomato, cantaloupe, potatoes, leafy greens.
HERBAL SOURCES OF	Rose hips, yellow dock root, raspberry leaf, red clover, hops, nettles, pine needles, dandelion greens, alfalfa, echinacea, skullcap, parsley, cayenne, paprika.
DEPLETED BY	Antibiotics, aspirin and other pain relievers, coffee, stress, aging, smoking, baking soda, high fever.

VITAMIN/MINERAL	**Vitamin D.**
FOUND IN	Fortified milk, butter, leafy green vegetables, egg yolk, fish oils, butter, liver, skin exposure to sunlight, shrimp.
HERBAL SOURCES OF	None; not found in plants.
DEPLETED BY	Mineral oil used on the skin, frequent baths, sunscreens with SPF 8 or higher.

VITAMIN/MINERAL	**Vitamin E.**
FOUND IN	Nuts, seeds, whole grains, fish-liver oils, fresh leafy greens, kale, cabbage, asparagus.
HERBAL SOURCES OF	Alfalfa, rose hips, nettles, Dang Gui, watercress, dandelions, seaweeds, wild seeds.
DEPLETED BY	Mineral oil, sulphates.

VITAMIN/MINERAL	**Vitamin K.**
FOUND IN	Leafy greens, corn and soybean oils, liver, cereals, dairy products, meats, fruits, egg yolk, blackstrap molasses.
HERBAL SOURCES OF	Nettles, alfalfa, kelp, green tea.
DEPLETED BY	X-rays, radiation, air pollution, enemas, frozen foods, antibiotics, rancid fats, aspirin.

Vitamin/Mineral	**Thiamine (vitamin B$_1$).**
Found In	Asparagus, cauliflower, cabbage, kale, spirulina, seaweeds, citrus.
Herbal Sources Of	Peppermint, burdock, sage, yellow dock, alfalfa, red clover, fenugreek, raspberry leaves, nettles, catnip, watercress, yarrow, briar rose buds, rose hips.
Depleted By	Caffeine, alcohol, stress, antibiotics.

Vitamin/Mineral	**Riboflavin (B$_2$).**
Found In	Beans, greens, onions, seaweeds, spirulina, dairy products, mushrooms.
Herbal Sources Of	Peppermint, alfalfa, parsley, echinacea, yellow dock, hops; dandelion, ginseng, dulse, kelp, fenugreek.
Depleted By	Caffeine, alcohol, stress, antibiotics.

Vitamin/Mineral	**Folic acid (B factor).**
Found In	Liver, eggs, leafy greens, yeast, legumes, whole grains, nuts, fruits (bananas, orange juice, grapefruit juice), vegetables (broccoli, spinach, aspargus, brussels sprouts).
Herbal Sources Of	Nettles, alfalfa, parsley, sage, catnip, peppermint, plantain, comfrey leaves, chickweed.
Depleted By	Alcohol, stress, antibiotics.

VITAMIN/MINERAL	**Niacin (B factor).**
FOUND IN	Grains, meats, and nuts, and especially asparagus, spirulina, cabbage, bee pollen.
HERBAL SOURCES OF	Hops, raspberry leaf, red clover, slippery elm, echinacea, licorice, rose hips, nettles, alfalfa, parsley.
DEPLETED BY	Alcohol, stress, antibiotics.

VITAMIN/MINERAL	**Bioflavonoids.**
FOUND IN	Citrus pulp and rind.
HERBAL SOURCES OF	Buckwheat greens, blue green algae, elderberries, hawthorn fruits, rose hips, horsetail, shepherd's purse.
DEPLETED BY	Nicotine, caffeine, alcohol.

VITAMIN/MINERAL	**Carotenes.**
FOUND IN	Carrots, cabbage, winter squash, sweet potatoes, dark leafy greens, apricots, spirulina, seaweeds.
HERBAL SOURCES OF	Peppermint, yellow dock, uva ursi, parsley, alfalfa, raspberry leaves, nettles, dandelion greens, kelp, green onions, violet leaves, cayenne, paprika, lamb's quarters, sage, peppermint, chickweed, horsetail, black cohosh, rose hips.
DEPLETED BY	Nicotine, caffeine, alcohol.

VITAMIN/MINERAL	**Essential fatty acids (EFAs), including GLA, omega-6, and omega-3.**
FOUND IN	Safflower oil, wheat germ oil, flaxseed seed oil, evening primrose, black current, borage.
HERBAL SOURCES OF	All wild plants.
DEPLETED BY	Nicotine, caffeine, alcohol.

VITAMIN/MINERAL	**Boron.**
FOUND IN	Organic fruits, vegetables, nuts.
HERBAL SOURCES OF	All organic weeds including chickweed, purslane, nettles, dandelion, yellow dock.
DEPLETED BY	Nicotine, caffeine, alcohol.

VITAMIN/MINERAL	**Calcium.**
FOUND IN	Milk and dairy products, leafy greens, broccoli, clams, oysters, almonds, walnuts, sunflower seeds, sesame seeds (e.g., tahini), legumes, tofu, softened bones of canned fish (sardines mackerel, salmon), seaweed vegetables, whole grain, whey, shellfish.
HERBAL SOURCES OF	Valerian, kelp, nettles, horsetail, peppermint, sage, uva ursi, yellow dock chickweed, red clover, oatstraw, parsley, blackcurrant leaf, raspberry leaf, plantain leaf/ seed, borage, dandelion leaf, amaranth leaves, lamb's quarter.
DEPLETED BY	Coffee, sugar, salt, alcohol, cortisone, enemas, too much phosphorus.

VITAMIN/MINERAL	**Chromium.**
FOUND IN	Barley grass, bee pollen, prunes, nuts, mushrooms, liver, beets, whole wheat.
HERBAL SOURCES OF	Oatstraw, nettles, red clover, catnip, dulse, wild yam, yarrow, horsetail, black cohosh, licorice, echinacea, valerian, sarsaparilla.
DEPLETED BY	White sugar.

VITAMIN/MINERAL	**Copper.**
FOUND IN	Liver, shellfish, nuts, legumes, water, organically grown grains, leafy greens, seaweeds, bittersweet chocolate.
HERBAL SOURCES OF	Skullcap, sage, horsetail, chickweed.
DEPLETED BY	Nicotine, caffeine, alcohol.

VITAMIN/MINERAL	**Heme Iron.** (Heme iron is easily absorbed by the body; non-heme iron not as easily absorbed, so should be taken with Vitamin C.)
FOUND IN	Liver, meat, poultry (non-heme iron: dried fruit, seeds, almonds, cashews, enriched and whole grains, legumes, green leafy vegetables).

Heme Iron. (continued)

HERBAL SOURCES OF   Chickweed, kelp, burdock, catnip,
                     horsetail, Althea root, milk thistle
                     seed, uva ursi, dandelion leaf/
                     root, yellow dock root, Dang Gui,
                     black cohosh, echinacea, plantain
                     leaves, sarsaparilla, nettles,
                     peppermint, licorice, valerian,
                     fenugreek.

DEPLETED BY   Coffee, black tea, enemas, alcohol,
                     aspirin, carbonated drinks, lack of
                     protein, too much dairy.

VITAMIN/MINERAL   **Magnesium.**

FOUND IN   Leafy greens, seaweeds, nuts, whole
                     grains, yogurt, cheese, potatoes,
                     corn, peas, squash.

HERBAL SOURCES OF   Oatstraw, licorice, kelp, nettle,
                     dulse, burdock, chickweed,
                     Althea root, horsetail, sage,
                     raspberry leaf, red clover,
                     valerian yellow dock, dandelion,
                     carrot tops, parsley, evening
                     primrose.

DEPLETED BY   Hot flashes, night sweats, crying jags,
                     alcohol, chemical diuretics,
                     enemas, antibiotics, excessive fat
                     intake.

VITAMIN/MINERAL	**Manganese.**
FOUND IN	Any leaf or seed from a plant grown in healthy soil, seaweeds.
HERBAL SOURCES OF	Raspberry leaf, uva ursi, chickweed, milk thistle, yellow dock, ginseng, wild yam, hops, catnip, echinacea, horsetail, kelp, nettles, dandelion.
DEPLETED BY	Nicotine, caffeine, alcohol.

VITAMIN/MINERAL	**Molybdenum.**
FOUND IN	Organically raised dairy products, legumes, grains, leafy greens.
HERBAL SOURCES OF	Nettles, dandelion greens, sage, oatstraw, fenugreek, raspberry leaves, red clover, horsetail, chickweed, seaweeds.
DEPLETED BY	Nicotine, caffeine, alcohol.

VITAMIN/MINERAL	**Nickel.**
FOUND IN	Chocolate, nuts, dried beans, cereals.
HERBAL SOURCES OF	Alfalfa, red clover, oatstraw, fenugreek.
DEPLETED BY	Nicotine, caffeine, alcohol.

VITAMIN/MINERAL	**Phosphorus.**
FOUND IN	Whole grains, seeds, nuts.
HERBAL SOURCES OF	Peppermint, yellow dock, milk thistle, fennel, hops, chickweed, nettles, dandelion, parsley, dulse, red clover.
DEPLETED BY	Antacids.

VITAMIN/MINERAL	**Potassium.**
FOUND IN	Celery, cabbage, peas, parsley, broccoli, peppers, carrots, potato skins, eggplant, whole grains, pears, citrus, seaweeds.
HERBAL SOURCES OF	Sage, catnip, hops, dulse, skullcap, peppermint, red clover, horsetail, kelp, nettles, borage, plantain.
DEPLETED BY	Frequent hot flashes with sweating, night sweats, coffee, sugar, salt, alcohol, enemas, vomiting, diarrhea, chemical diuretics, dieting.

VITAMIN/MINERAL	**Selenium.**
FOUND IN	Dairy products, seaweeds, grains, garlic, liver, kidneys, fish, shellfish.
HERBAL SOURCES OF	Catnip, milk thistle, valerian, dulse, black cohosh, ginseng, uva ursi, hops, echinacea, kelp, raspberry leaf, rose buds and hips, hawthorn berries, fenugreek, sarsaparilla, yellow dock.
DEPLETED BY	Nicotine, caffeine, alcohol, mercury, excess Vitamin C, excess iron.

VITAMIN/MINERAL	**Silicon.**
FOUND IN	Unrefined grains, root vegetables, spinach, leeks.
HERBAL SOURCES OF	Horsetail, dulse, echinacea, cornsilk, burdock, oatstraw, licorice, chickweed, uva ursi, sarsaparilla.
DEPLETED BY	Nicotine, caffeine, alcohol.

VITAMIN/MINERAL	**Sulfur.**
FOUND IN	Eggs, dairy products, cabbage family plants, onions, garlic, parsley, watercress.
HERBAL SOURCES OF	Nettles, sage, plantain, horsetail.
DEPLETED BY	Nicotine, caffeine, alcohol.

VITAMIN/MINERAL	**Zinc.**
FOUND IN	Oysters, seafood, meat, liver, eggs, whole grains, wheat germ, pumpkin seeds, spirulina.
HERBAL SOURCES OF	Skullcap, sage, wild yam, chickweed, echinacea, nettles, dulse, milk thistle, sarsaparilla.
DEPLETED BY	Alcohol and air pollution.

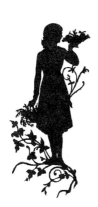

Links from *sarahealth.com*

For more information about disease prevention and wellness, visit me online at *www.sarahealth.com,* where you will find more than 300 links—including those noted here—related to your good health and wellness.

Abbott Laboratories: *www.abbott.com*

About.com (Diabetes):
diabetes.about.com.health/diabetes/mbody.htm

American Diabetes Association: *www.diabetes.org*

American Association of Clinical Endocrinologists:
www.aace.com

Amputation Prevention Global Resource Center
(prevention, causes, signs and symptoms, and treatment
information): *www.diabetesresource.com*

Bayer Corp: *www.glucometer.com/product.htm*

Blindness and Diabetes Resource and Support (includes back
issues of the "Voice of the Diabetic" from the National
Federation of the Blind): *www.prevent-blindness.org*

Canadian Diabetes Association: *www.diabetes.ca*

Canadian National Institute for the Blind: *www.cnib.ca*

Canadian Organic Growers Association: *www.cog.ca*

Chronimed Inc: *www.chronimed.com*

Diabetes.com (Diabetes and Sexual Intimacy; award-winning site with health library, products and prescriptions, newsroom): *www.diabetes.com/site/*

Diabetic Gourmet Magazine (free newsletter, daily tidbits, menus, and forum): *gourmetconnection.com/diabetic/*

Diabetes mall (targets both a general audience and medical professionals; information about research, prevention, and education; support group): *www.diabetesnet.com/index.html*

Diabetes monitor (a great source of patient information, research, statistics, and education; includes registry of links): *www.diabetesmonitor.com*

Diabetes Type II Resource and Discussion Page (information specific to those with Type 2 Diabetes): *home.ptd.net/~hwagner/2r.htm*

Diabetes Type 2 (from the American Medical Association; symptoms, screening, diagnosis, complications, etc.): *www.ama-assn.org/insight/spe_con/diabetes.htm*

HealthNet-Diabetes (treatment, patient education, advice): *www.healthnet.com*

The Islet Foundation (foundation dedicated to finding a cure for insulin-dependent diabetes; interesting resources and information on the future of diabetes): *www.islet.org*

The Kidney Foundation of Canada: *www.kidney.ca*

Life Scan Inc: *www.lifescan.com* (United States) *www.lifescan-can.com* (Canada)

LXN Corp: *www.lxncorp.com*

Managing your Diabetes (official site of Eli Lilly & Co.; lots of great information about diabetes products): *diabetes.lilly.com*

Medic Alert (site of the trademarked Medic Alert emblem): *www.medicalert.org*

Medic Alert: *www.medicalert.ca*

National Diabetes Fact Sheet (from the U.S. Center for Disease Control and Prevention): *www.cdc.gov/diabetes*

National Diabetes Information Clearinghouse (and Diabetes database): *www.niddk.nih.gov/NDIC/NDIC.html*

National Institute of Diabetes and Digestive Kidney Disease: *www.niddk.nih.gov/*

NutraSweet (facts about this artificial sugar substitute): *www.alaskanet:/80/~tne/*

Olestra (information about this synthetic fat product now available in the United States): *www.diabetesmonitor.com/olestra.htm*

Polymer Tech Systems Inc: *www.diabetes-testing.com*

QuestStar Medical Inc: *www.queststarmedical.com*

Recipe of the Day (features a new healthy recipe every day, Monday through Thursday; from the ADA): *www.diabetes.org/ada/rcptoday.html*

The Roche Group (Accu-Check): *www.roche.com*

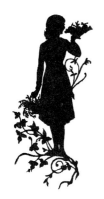

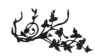

Bibliography

"Acarbose (Prandase)." *New Drugs/ Drug News,* Ontario College of Pharmacists Drug Information Service Newsletter, Vol. 14, No. 2 (March/April 1996).

The Accu-Chek Advantage System. Patient information. Eli Lilly of Canada Inc., distributed 1997.

"The Ad Hoc Technical Committee Working Group on Development of Management Principles and Guidelines for Subsistence Catches of Whales by Indigenous (Aboriginal) Peoples." *International Whaling Commission and Aboriginal/Subsistence Whaling: April 1979 to July 1981.* Special Issue 4, International Whaling Commission, Cambridge, England.

"Advocacy in Action." *Diabetes Dialogue,* Vol. 43, No. 3 (Fall 1996).

"The Agony of De-Feet." *Equilibrium*, Issue 1 (1996): 12–14.

"AHA Stroke Connection." Patient information retrieved online July 2001 from the American Heart Association (*www.americanheart.org*).

Alcohol and Diabetes—Do They Mix? Booklet. Canadian Diabetes Association, distributed 1996.

Ali, Elvis, et al. *Natural Remedies and Supplments: The All In One Guide Niagara Falls.* New York: Ages Publications, 1999.

Allard, Johane P. Excerpts from "International Conference on Antioxidant Vitamins and Beta-Carotene in Disease Prevention: A Canadian Perspective," 1996.

Allardice, Pamela. Essential Oils: The Fragrant Art of Aromatherapy. Vancouver: Raincoast Books, 1999.

Allsop, Karen F., and Janette Brand Miller. "Honey Revisited: A Reappraisal of Honey in Preindustrial Diets." *British Journal of Nutrition,* Vol. 75 (1996): 513–520.

American Board for Certification in Orthotics and Prosthetics Inc. Retrieved online July 2001 from the Amputee Web Site (*www.amputee-online.ca*).

American Diabetes Association. "An Introduction to Oral Medications for Diabetes." Posted to *Diabetes.com.* January 1999.

——. "Standards of Medical Care for Patients with Diabetes Mellitus." *Diabetes Care,* Vol. 21, Supp. 1, Clinical Practice Recommendations, 1998.

——. "The United Kingdom Prospective Diabetes Study (UKPDS) for Type 2 Diabetes: What You Need to Know About the Results of a Long-Term Study." Posted to *www.diabetes.org.* January, 1999.

——. Online information. Document ID: ADA035, 1995.

Amputation Prevention Global Resource Center. *Prevent Foot Ulcers and Amputations.* Booklet. Retrieved from *www.diabetesrousource.com.* July 2001.

Anderson, Pauline. "Researchers Predict 'Beginning of the End' of Diabetes." *The Medical Post* (August 22, 1995).

The Antioxidant Connection: Visiting Speakers Discuss Immunity, Diabetes. Published by the Vitamin Information Program of Hoffman-La Roche Ltd., September 1995.

Armstrong, David G., Lawrence A. Lavery, and Lawrence B. Harkless. "Treatment-Based Classification System for Assessment and Care of Diabetic Feet." *Journal of the American Podiatric Medical Association*, Vol. 87, No. 7 (July 1996): 303–308.

Balancing Your Blood Sugar: A Guide for People with Diabetes. Patient information. Canadian Diabetes Association, distributed 1997.

"Bayer Launches Major International Research Project into Prevention of Diabetes." Media Release, March 5, 1997.

Beck, Leslie, R.D. *Leslie Beck's Nutrition Guide for Women.* Toronto: Penguin Books, 2001.

Bell, S.J., and R.A. Forse. "Nutritional Management of Hypoglycemia." *Diabetes Education*, Vol. 25, No. 1 (Jan–Feb 1999): 41–47.

Bequaert Holmes, Helen, and Laura M. Purdy, eds. *Feminist Perspectives in Medical Ethics.* Bloomington: Indiana University Press, 1992.

Berndl, Leslie. "Understanding Fat." *Diabetes Dialogue*, Vol. 42, No. 1 (Spring 1995): 17–20.

Beyers, Joanne. "How Sweet It Is!" *Diabetes Dialogue*, Vol. 42, No. 1 (Spring 1995): 6–8.

Biermann, June, and Barbara Toohey. *The Diabetic's Book.* New York: Perigee Books, 1992.

Blood Glucose Monitoring: Guidelines to a Healthier You. Patient information from Bayer Inc. Healthcare Division, distributed 1997.

"Blood Pressure: Check It Out." *Countdown USA: Countdown to a Healthy Heart*, Allegheny General Hospital and Voluntary Hospitals of America, Inc., 1990.

Blood Sugar Testing Diary. Patient information. Becton Dickinson Consumer Products, 1996.

Bonen, Arent. "Fueling Your Tank." *Diabetes Dialogue*, Vol. 42, No. 4 (Winter 1995): 13–16.

Bril, Vera. "Diabetic Neuropathy—Can It Be Treated?" *Diabetes Dialogue*, Vol. 41, No. 4 (Winter 1994): 8–9.

British Columbia Women's Community Consultation Report. *The Challenges Ahead for Women's Health.* Vancouver: B.C. Women's Hospital and Health Centre Society, Vancouver, 1995.

Bureau of Human Prescription Drugs, Drugs Directorate, Health Protection Branch, Health Canada. *Drugs Directorate Guidelines, Directions for Use of Estrogen-Progestin Combination Oral Contraceptives.* Ottawa: Bureau of Human Prescription Drugs, 1994.

"Buying Your Prosthesis." Retrieved online July 2001 from the Amputee Web Site (*www.amputee-online.ca*).

Canadian Diabetes Association. "Guidelines for the Nutritional Management of Diabetes Mellitus in the New Millennium." A position statement. Reprinted from *Canadian Journal Diabetes Care*, Vol. 23, No. 3 (2000): 56–69.

——. "Health...the Smoke-Free Way." *Equilibrium*, Issue 1 (1996): 1–4.

Canadian Medical Association Journal and the Canadian Diabetes Association. "1998 Clinical Practice Guidelines for the Management of Diabetes in Canada." Supplement to *CMAJ*, Vol. 159, No. 8, Suppl. (1998): s1–s27.

Canadian Task Force on the Periodic Health Examination. *The Canadian Guide to Clinical Preventive Health Care.* Ottawa: Health Canada, 1994.

"Canons of Ethical Conduct for Prosthetists." March 1997, Committee on Professional Discipline. Retrieved online from The Amputee Web Site (*www.amputee-online.ca*). July 2001.

"Carbohydrate Counting: A New Way to Plan Meals." American Diabetes Association. Posted to *Diabetes.com*. January 1999.

Cattral, Mark. "Pancreas Transplantation." *Diabetes Dialogue*, Vol. 43, No. 4 (Winter 1996): 6–8.

Chaddock, Brenda. "Activity Is Key to Diabetes Health." *Canadian Pharmacy Journal* (March 1997): 45.

——. "Blood-Glucose Testing: Keep Up with the Trend." *Canadian Pharmacy Journal* (September 1996): 17.

——. "Doing the Things That Make a Difference." *Canadian Pharmacy Journal* (July/August 1996): 19.

——. "The Right Way to Read a Label." *Canadian Pharmacy Journal* (May 1996): 26.

——. "Foul Weather Fitness: The Hardest Part Is Getting Started." *Canadian Pharmacy Journal* (March 1996): 42.

——. "The Magic of Exercise." *Canadian Pharmacy Journal* (September 1995): 45.

The Challenge: Newsletter of the International Diabetic Athletes Association Vol. XI, No. I (Spring 1997): 1–2.

"Choosing Your Sweetener." Product information. PROSWEET Canada, 1997.

Christrup, Janet. "Nuts About Nuts: The Joys of Growing Nut Trees." *Cognition* (July 1991): 20–22.

Clarke, Bill. "Action Figures." *Diabetes Dialogue*, Vol. 43, No. 3 (Fall 1996): 14–16.

Clarke, Peter V. "Hemoglobin A1c Test Helps Long-Term Diabetes Management." *Monitor*, Vol. 1, No. 1 (1996): 1–3. Medisense Canada Inc.

Cleave, Barbara. "Viewpoint." *Diabetes Dialogue*, Vol. 44, No. 2 (Summer 1997): 2.

"Complications: The Long-Term Picture." *Equilibrium*, Issue 1 (1996): 8–10. Canadian Diabetes Association.

Cronier, Claire. "Sweetest Choices." *Diabetes Dialogue*, Vol. 44, No. 1 (Spring 1997): 26–27.

Cunningham, John J. "Vitamins, Minerals and Diabetes." Excerpted from Canadian Diabetes Association Conference, 1995.

"Dental Care." Retrieved online from the Canadian Dental Association (*www.cda.adc.caww*). July 2001.

Deutsch, Nancy. "Vitamin C Stores Critical for Diabetics." *Family Practice*, 11 (November 1996): 24.

Dextrolog: For Recording Blood and Urine Glucose Test Results. Booklet. Bayer Inc. Healthcare Division, distributed 1997.

Diabetes and Kidney Disease. Patient information. The Kidney Foundation of Canada, 1995.

"Diabetes and Kidney Disease." Retrieved online from the Kidney Foundation of Canada (*www.kidney.ca*). July 2001.

Diabetes and Non-Prescription Drugs: Guidelines to a Healthier You. Patient information. Bayer Inc. Healthcare Division, distributed 1997.

"Diabetes and the Eye." Retrieved online July 2001 from the Blindness and Visual Impairment Centre, Canadian National Institute for the Blind www.cnib.ca.

Diabetes Education. Patient information. Canadian Diabetes Association, distributed 1997.

"Diabetes Implants Tested." *Los Angeles Daily News* (Jan. 23, 1997).

"Diabetes Raises Dementia Risk." Reuters (Feb. 13, 1997).

Diabetes. Patient information. Pharma Plus, distributed 1997.

"Diabetes: An Undetected Time-Bomb." *CARP News* (April 1996): 12.

"Diabetes: Facts and Figures." *News from the VIP*, No. 2 (Fall 1995): 1. Vitamin Information Program, Fine Chemicals Division of Hoffman-La Roche Ltd.

"Diabetes: What Is It?" *Equilibrium*, Canadian Diabetes Association, Issue 1 (1996): 1–4.

"Diets Slow Reaction Times." Reuters (April 8, 1997).

"Double Trouble." *Countdown USA: Countdown to a Healthy Heart*. Allegheny General Hospital and Voluntary Hospitals of America, Inc., 1990.

Doyle, Patricia. "Insulin—The Facts." Canadian Diabetes Association, 1995.

Drum, David, and Terry Zierenberg. *The Type 2 Diabetes Sourcebook*. Los Angeles: Lowell House, 1998.

Dutcher, Lisa. "A Wholistic Approach to Diabetes Management." *Diabetes Dialogue*, Vol. 41, No. 3 (Fall 1994): 42.

Engel, June. "Eating Fibre." *Diabetes Dialogue*, Vol. 44, No. 1 (Spring 1997): 16–18.

———. "Beyond Vitamins: Phytochemicals to Help Fight Disease." *Health News*, Vol. 14 (June 1996): 1.

Exercise: Guidelines to a Healthier You. Patient information. Bayer Inc. Healthcare Division, distributed 1997.

The Expert Committee on the Diagnosis and Classification of Diabetes Mellitus. *Report of the Expert Committee on the Diagnosis and Classification of Diabetes Mellitus,* American Diabetes Association, January 1, 1998.

Farquhar, Andrew. "Exercising Essentials." *Diabetes Dialogue*, Vol. 43, No. 3 (Fall 1996): 6–8.

"The Fat Trap." *Countdown USA: Countdown to a Healthy Heart*. Allegheny General Hospital and Voluntary Hospitals of America, Inc., 1990.

"FDA Approves Drug to Reduce Insulin Needs for Some Diabetics." The Associated Press (Jan. 30, 1997).

Findlay, Deborah, and Leslie Miller. "Medical Power and Women's Bodies." In B.S. Bolaria and R. Bolaria, eds., *Women, Medicine and Health*. Halifax: Fernwood, 1994.

"Flick Your Risk: By Tossing Out Those Cigarettes, You Can Slash Your Chances of Heart Disease." *Countdown USA: Countdown to a Healthy Heart*, Allegheny General Hospital and Voluntary Hospitals of America, Inc., 1990.

"Folic Acid Surveys Say Consumer Awareness Is Low." *News from the VIP*, No. 2 (Fall 1995): 1–2. Vitamin Information Program, Fine Chemicals Division of Hoffman-La Roche Ltd.

"Following the Patient with Chronic Disease." *Patient Care Canada*, Vol. 7, No. 5 (May 1996): 22–38.

"Following the Patient With Stable Chronic Disease: Type II Diabetes Mellitus." *Patient Care Canada*, Vol. 7, No. 5 (May 1996): 22–41.

——. "Nutrient Claims Guide for Individual Foods." Special Report, Focus on Food Labeling. FDA Publication no. 95-2289.

Food and Exercise: Guidelines to a Healthier You. Patient information. Bayer Inc. Healthcare Division, distributed 1997.

"Foot Care and Ulcer Prevention for People with Diabetes: Is Amputation the Only Answer?" Retrieved online from the University of Manitoba (*www.umanitoba.ca/*) Diabetes Research & Treatment Centre. July 2001.

Fraser, Elizabeth, and Bill Clarke. "Loafing Around." *Diabetes Dialogue*, Vol. 44, No. 1 (Spring 1997): 32–33.

Gabrys, Jennifer. "Ask the Professionals." *Diabetes Dialogue*, Vol. 43, No. 4 (Winter 1996): 60–61.

Get the Best Out of Life. Patient information. Canadian Diabetes Association, distributed 1997.

Getting to the Roots of a Vegetarian Diet. Baltimore: Vegetarian Resource Group, 1997.

Graham, Peg. "Rising Expectations." *Diabetes Dialogue*, Vol. 44, No. 2 (Summer 1997): 32–33.

Gregson, Ian. "An Amputee's Perspective." Retrieved online from The Amputee Web Site (*www.amputee-online.ca*). July 2001.

"Grieving Necessary to Accept Diabetes." *Diabetes Dialogue*, Vol. 41, No. 3 (Fall 1994): 35–36.

"The Gum Disease Project." Retrieved from *www.periodiabetes.com*. July 2001.

Guthrie, Diana, and Richard A. Guthrie. *The Diabetes Sourcebook*. Los Angeles: Lowell House, 1996.

Harrison, Pam. "Rethinking Obesity." *Family Practice* (March 11, 1996): 24.

"Heart and Stroke Foundation's Annual Report Card." Retrieved online from the Heart and Stroke Foundation of Canada (*www.na.heartandstroke.ca/*). July 2001.

Heart and Stroke Foundation of Canada. *The Canadian Family Guide to Stroke: Prevention, Treatment, Recovery*. Toronto: Random House, 1996.

"Heart Attack No Stranger to Canadians." Retrieved online from the Heart and Stroke Foundation of Canada (*www.na.heartandstroke.ca/*). July 2001.

"Heart Attack Picture in Canada Receives Mixed Grade." Retrieved online from the Heart and Stroke Foundation of Canada (*www.na.heartandstroke.ca/*). February 7, 2001.

"Heart Attack Survival in Canada." Retrieved online from the Heart and Stroke Foundation of Canada (*www.na.heartandstroke.ca/*). July 2001.

Heart Disease and Stroke. Patient information. The Heart and Stroke Foundation of Ontario, distributed 1997.

"The Heart Healthy Kitchen." *Countdown USA: Countdown to a Healthy Heart.* Allegheny General Hospital and Voluntary Hospitals of America, Inc., 1990.

"Hemodialysis." Retrieved online from the Kidney Foundation of Canada (*www.kidney.ca*). July 2001.

High Blood Pressure and Your Kidneys. Patient information. The Kidney Foundation of Canada, 1995.

"High-Carbohydrate Diet Not for Everyone." Reuters (April 16, 1997).

Higley, Connie, Alan Higley, Pat Leatham, *Aromatherapy A-Z.* Carlsbad, Calif.: Hay House, 1998.

Ho, Marian. "Learning Your ABCs, Part Two." *Diabetes Dialogue*, Vol. 43, No. 3 (Fall 1996): 38–40.

Hommel, Cynthia Abbott. "The SUGAR Group." *Diabetes Dialogue*, Vol. 41, No. 3 (Fall 1994): 21–23.

"Hostility and Heart Risk." Reuters Health Summary (April 22, 1997).

"How Adults Are Learning to Manage Diabetes with Their Lifestyle." *The Globe and Mail* (November 1, 1996).

How Do I Choose a Healthy Diet? Patient information. The Heart and Stroke Foundation of Ontario, distributed 1997.

How to Choose Your New Blood Glucose Meter. Patient information. LifeScan Canada Inc., distributed 1997.

How to Cope with a Brief Illness: A Guide for the Person Taking Insulin. Patient information. The Canadian Diabetes Association, March 1996.

How to Take Insulin. Patient information. Monoject Diabetes Care Products, distributed 1997.

Hunt, John A. "Fueling Up." *Diabetes Dialogue*, Vol. 41, No. 4 (Winter 1994): 20–21.

Hunter, J.E., and T.H. Applewhite. "Reassessment of Trans Fatty Acid Availability in the U.S. Diet." *American Journal of Clinical Nutrition*, 54 (1991): 363–369.

Hurley, Jane, and Stephen Schmidt. "Going with the Grain." *Nutrition Action* (October 1994): 10–11.

IFIC Review: Intense Sweeteners: Effects on Appetite and Weight Management. International Food Information Council, 1100 Connecticut Avenue N.W., Suite 430, Washington D.C. 20036, November 1995.

IFIC Review: Uses and Nutritional Impact of Fat Reduction Ingredients. International Food Information Council 1100 Connecticut Avenue N.W., Suite 430, Washington D.C. 20036, October 1995.

"The Importance of Braille Literacy." Retrieved online from the Blindness and Visual Impairment Centre, Canadian National Institute for the Blind (*www.cnib.ca*). July 2001.

"Improving Treatment Outcomes in NIDDM: The Questions and Controversies." *The Diabetes Report*, Issue 1, Vol. 2 (1996): 1–2.

"Increased Awareness of Stroke Symptoms Could Dramatically Reduce Stroke Disability—New NIH Public Education Campaign Says Bystanders Can Play Key Role." (May 8, 2001) Retrieved online from the American Heart Association (*www.americanheart.org*).

"Insulin and Type 2 Diabetes."*Equilibrium*, Issue 1 (1996): 29–30.

Insulin Management Information. Patient information from Eli Lilly and Co., distributed 1997.

Jovanovic-Peterson, Lois, June Biermann, and Barbara Toohey. *The Diabetic Woman: All Your Questions Answered.* New York: G.P. Putnam's Sons, 1996.

Joyce, Carol. "What's New in Type 2." *Diabetes Dialogue*, Vol. 43, No. 3 (Fall 1996): 32–36, 63.

Kalla, Timothy B. "Complications: Footcare and the Trouble with Ulcers." Retrieved online from the Canadian Diabetes Association (*www.diabetes.ca*). July 2001.

Kaptchuk, Ted, and Micheal Croucher. *The Healing Arts: A Journal Through the Faces of Medicine*. London: The British Broadcasting Corporation, 1986.

Kelly, Catherine. "Hormone Replacement Therapy." *Diabetes Dialogue*, Vol. 44, No. 2 (Summer 1997): 28–30.

Kermode-Scott, Barbara. "NIDDM Affecting Huge Numbers, Says Expert." *Family Practice* (March 11, 1996): 21.

Ketone Testing: Guidelines to a Healthier You. Patient information. Bayer Inc. Healthcare Division, distributed 1997.

Khan, Gabriel M., and Henry J.L. Marriot. *Heart Trouble Encyclopedia*. Toronto: Stoddart, 1996.

Kidney Stones. Patient information. The Kidney Foundation of Canada, distributed 1995.

Kra, J. Siegfried. *What Every Woman Must Know About Heart Disease* New York: Warner Books, 1996.

Kuczmarski, R.J., et al. "Increasing Prevalence of Overweight Among U.S. Adults: The National Health and Nutrition Examination Surveys, 1960 to 1991." *Journal of the American Medical Association*, 272 (1994): 205–211.

Kushi, Mishio. *The Cancer Prevention Guide.* New York: St. Martin's Press, 1993.

Lad, Dr. Vasant. Ayurveda: the Science of Self-Healing. Santa Fe, N.M.: Lotus Press: 1984.

Leiter, Lawrence A. "Acarbose: New Treatment in NIDDM Patients." *New Drugs/Drug News*, Vol. 14, No. 2 (1997). Ontario College of Pharmacists.

Levine, R.J. *Ethics and Regulation of Clinical Research*. New Haven, Conn.: Yale University Press, 1988.

Lichtenstein, A.H., et al. "Hydrogenation Impairs the Hypolipidemic Effect of Corn Oil in Humans." *Arteriosclerosis and Thrombosis*, 13 (1993): 154–161.

Lichti, Janice C. "Mind Boosters." *Healing Arts Magazine* (March 1996): 14–15.

Liebman, Bonnie. "Syndrome X: The Risks of High Insulin." *Nutrition Action*, Vol. 27, No. 2 (March 2000): 3–8.

Linden, Ron. "Hyperbaric Medicine." *Diabetes Dialogue*, Vol. 43, No. 4 (Fall 1996): 24–26.

Lindsay, J.E. "Multiple Pain Complaints in Amputees." *Journal of Rehabilitation and Social Medicine*, Vol. 78 (1985): 452–455.

Little, Linda. "Vitamin E May Help Cut Diabetics' Risk of Heart Disease." *The Medical Post* (May 14, 1996): 5.

Little, Margaret. "Step Right Up." *Diabetes Dialogue*, Vol. 43, No. 3 (Fall 1996).

Living Well. Patient information. Canadian Diabetes Association, distributed 1997.

"Low Blood Sugars: Your Questions Answered." *Equilibrium*, Issue 1 (1996): 31–32.

Macdonald, Jeanette. "The Facts About Menopause." *Diabetes Dialogue*, Volume 44, No. 2 (Summer 1997): 24–26.

Marshall, M., E. Helmes, and A.B. Deathe. "A Comparison of Psychosocial Functioning and Personality in Amputee and Chronic Pain Patients." *Clinical Journal of Pain* 8 (1992): 351–357.

Mastroianni, Anna C., Ruth Faden and Daniel Federman, eds. *Women and Health Research: Ethical and Legal Issues of Including Women in Clinical Studies*, Vol. 1. Washington: National Academy Press, 1994.

Mature Lifestyles: High Blood Pressure. Patient information. Health Watch/Shoppers Drug Mart, distributed 1997.

MediSense Blood Glucose Sensor. Product monograph, 1995.

Micral-S Kidney Chek. Patient information. Eli Lilly of Canada/ Boehringer Mannheim Canada Inc., distributed 1997.

"Monitoring Your Blood Sugar." *Equilibrium*, Issue 1 (1996): 33.

Musgrove, Lorraine. "Ask the Professionals." *Diabetes Dialogue*, Vol. 44, No. 1 (Spring 1997): 60–61.

National Kidney Foundation. *Dialysis.* Booklet. Retrieved online from *www.kidney.org.* July 2001.

——. *End Stage Renal Disease in the United States.* Booklet. Retrieved online from *www.kidney.org.* July 2001.

——. "Microalbuninuria in Diabetic Kidney Disease." Retrieved online from *www.kidney.org.* July 2001.

——. "Preventing Diabetic Kidney Disease." Retrieved online from *www.kidney.org.* July 2001.

"New Developments in the Management of Type II Diabetes." *The Diabetes Report*, Issue 2, Vol. 1 (1995): 1, 2.

"New Perspectives in the Management of NIDDM." *The Diabetes Report*, Issue 3, Vol. 1 (1996): 1, 3.

"New Tool Allows Early Prediction of Patient's Stroke Outcome." Retrieved online from the National Institute of Neurological Disorders and Stroke (*www.ninds.nih.gov*). June 28, 2001.

Non-Insulin Dependent Diabetes Mellitus. Patient information. National Pharmacy Continuing Education Program and Bayer Inc., distributed February 1997.

Nutrition for Diabetes. Patient information manual from Novo Nordisk Canada Inc., distributed 1996.

"Nutrition News." *Diabetes Dialogue*, Vol. 43, No. 4 (Winter 1996): 57.

"Nutrition News." *Diabetes Dialogue*, Vol. 44, No. 1 (Spring 1997): 56.

"Nutrition Principles for the Management of Diabetes and Related Complications (Technical Review)." *Diabetes Care*, Vol. 17 (1994): 490–518.

"Oats Are In." *Countdown USA: Countdown to a Healthy Heart*. Allegheny General Hospital and Voluntary Hospitals of America, Inc., 1990.

"Olestra: Yes or No? Excerpt from The University of California at Berkeley Wellness Letter." *Diabetes Dialogue*, Vol. 43, No. 3 (Fall 1996): 44.

One Touch Profile: For Complete Diabetes Management. Patient information. LifeScan Canada Inc., distributed 1997.

Orbach, Susie. *Fat Is a Feminist Issue.* New York: Berkley Books, 1990.

"Physical Activity." *Equilibrium*, Issue 1 (1996).

Poirier, Laurinda M., and Katharine M. Coburn. *Women and Diabetes: Life Planning for Health and Wellness.* New York: American Diabetes Association and Bantam Books, 1997.

"Position of the American Dietetic Association: Use of Nutritive and Nonnutritive Sweeteners." *Journal of the American Dietetic Association*, Vol. 93 (1993): 816–822.

Practical Advice for the Prandase Patient. Booklet. Bayer Inc. Healthcare Division, distributed 1996.

Preventing the Complications of Diabetes: Guidelines to a Healthier You. Patient information. Bayer Inc. Healthcare Division, distributed 1997.

"Prevention and Treatment of Obesity: Application to Type 2 Diabetes (Technical Review)." *Diabetes Care*, Vol. 20 (1997): 1744–1766.

Prochaska, James O. "A Revolution in Diabetes Evaluation." Excerpted from the Canadian Diabetes Association Conference, 1995.

"Proper Knowledge of a Healthy Diet Makes Huge Difference." *The Globe and Mail* (November 1, 1996): 3.

PROSWEET: The Low Calorie Pure Sugar Taste Sweetener. Product information. PROSWEET Canada, distributed 1997.

"Protein Content of the Diabetic Diet (Technical Review)." *Diabetes Care*, Vol. 17 (1994): 1502–1513.

"Putting Fun Back into Food." International Food Information Council, 1100 Connecticut Avenue N.W., Suite 430, Washington D.C. 20036, 1997.

"Q & A About Fatty Acids and Dietary Fats." International Food Information Council, 1100 Connecticut Avenue N.W., Suite 430, Washington D.C. 20036, 1997.

"Q & A on Low-Calorie Sweeteners." *The Diabetes News*, Vol. 1, Issue 2 (Spring 1997): 3.

Real World Factors That Interfere with Blood-Glucose Meter Accuracy. Patient information. MediSense Canada Inc., distributed 1996.

The Receptor Vol. 7, No. 3 (Fall/Winter 1996).

"Recovering After a Stroke." Retrieved online from the Agency for Healthcare Research and Quality (*www.ahrq.gov/*). July 2001.

Reddy, Sethu. "Smoking and Diabetes." *Diabetes Dialogue*, Vol. 42, No. 4 (Winter 1995): 33–35.

Reducing Your Risk of Diabetes Complications. Patient information. MediSense Canada Inc., distributed 1997.

Rosenthal, M. Sara. *The Type 2 Diabetic Woman*: New York: McGraw-Hill/Contemporary, 1999.

——. *50 Ways to Manage Stress:* New York: McGraw-Hill/ Contemporary, 2001.

——. *50 Ways Women Can Prevent Heart Disease* New York: McGraw-Hill/Contemporary, 2000.

Rosenthal, M. Sara. *50 Ways to Manage Type 2 Diabetes*. New York: McGraw-Hill/Contemporary, 2001.

——.*Managing PMS Naturally* Toronto: Penguin Books, 2001.

——.*Women Managing Stress* Toronto: Penguin Books, 2002.

——. *The Type 2 Diabetic Woman.* Chicago: NTC/ Contemporary, 1999.

Rowlands, Liz, and Denis Peter. "Diabetes—Yukon Style." *Diabetes Dialogue*, Vol. 41, No. 3 (Fall 1994).

Rubin, Alan L. *Diabetes for Dummies.* Chicago: IDG Books, 1999.

Ruggiero, Laura. *Helping People with Diabetes Change: Practical Applications of the Stages of Change Model.* Professional information. LifeScan Education Institute, distributed 1997.

Ryan, David. "At the Controls." *Diabetes Dialogue*, Vol. 43, No. 3 (Fall 1996): 20–21.

Safety First. Patient information. Becton Dickinson and Co. Canada Inc., distributed 1997.

Schwartz, Carol. "An Eye-Opener." *Diabetes Dialogue*, Vol. 43, No. 4 (Winter 1996): 20–22.

——. "Complications: Your Eyes and Diabetic Retinopathy." Retrieved online from the Canadian Diabetes Association (*www.diabetes.ca*). July 2001.

"Selected Vitamins and Minerals in Diabetes (Technical Review)." *Diabetes Care*, Vol. 17 (1994): 464–479.

Seto, Carol. "Nutrition Labelling—U.S. Style." *Diabetes Dialogue*, Vol. 42, No. 1 (Spring 1995): 32–34.

7 Key Factors for Real World Accuracy in the Real World. Patient information from MediSense Canada Inc., distributed 1997.

7 Key Steps to Control Your Diabetes. Patient information from MediSense Canada Inc., distributed 1997.

"Seven Tips for Your Sick Day Blues." *Equilibrium*, Issue 1 (1996): 38–41.

Sherwin, Susan. *Patient No Longer: Feminist Ethics and Health Care*. Philadelphia: Temple University Press, 1984.

Sinclair, A.J. "Rational Approaches to the Treatment of Patients with Non-insulin-Dependent Diabetes Mellitus." *Practical Diabetes Supplement*, Vol. 10, No. 6 (Nov./Dec. 1993): 515–520.

"Sorting Out the Facts About Fat." International Food Information Council, 1100 Connecticut Avenue N.W., Suite 430, Washington D.C. 20036, 1997.

Spicer, Kay. "Traditional Foods of Aboriginal Canadians." *Diabetes Dialogue*, Vol. 41, No. 3 (Fall 1994).

"Spring at Last!" *The Diabetes News,* prepared by the LifeScan Education Institute, Spring 1996.

Stehlin, Dori. "A Little Lite Reading" posted to FDA Web site (*www.fda.gov/fdac/foodlabel/diabetes.html*).

"Study: You Can Lose Weight and Cigarettes." Reuters (June 19, 1997).

Sucralose Overview. Product information from Splenda (brand sweetener) Information Centre, distributed 1997.

Surestep. Patient information. LifeScan Canada Inc, distributed 1997.

"Sweet Promise from Sugar Substitute?" *The Medical Post* (July 2, 1996): 55.

Taking Care of Your Feet: Guidelines to a Healthier You. Patient information. Bayer Inc., Healthcare Division, distributed 1997.

"10 Tips to Healthy Eating." American Dietetic Association and National Center for Nutrition and Dietetics (NCND), April 1994.

Tetley, Deborah. "Fish Farmer Hopes to Tame Diabetes on Akwesasne." *The Toronto Star* (April 12, 1997).

Thompson, John Herd, with Allen Singer. *Canada 1922–1939: Decades of Discord.* Toronto: McClelland & Stewart, Ltd., 1985.

Todd, Robert. "The Sporting Life." *Diabetes Dialogue*, Vol. 43, No. 4 (Fall 1996): 28–29.

Treating Kidney Failure. Patient information. The Kidney Foundation of Canada, distributed 1995.

Understanding Type 2 Diabetes: Guidelines for a Healthier You. Patient information. Bayer Inc. Healthcare Division, distributed 1997.

Urinary Tract Infections. Patient information from The Kidney Foundation of Canada, distributed 1995.

Utiger, Robert. "Restoring Fertility in Women with PCOS." *The New England Journal of Medicine*, Vol. 335, No. 9 (August 29, 1996).

Wanless, Melanie. "The Weight Debate." *Diabetes Dialogue*, Vol. 44, No. 1 (Spring 1997): 22–25.

Watch Your Step. Booklet. Norvo Nordisk Canada, Inc., distributed 1996.

"We're Winning: By Changing Lifestyles, We're Proving Every Day That Coronary Disease Can Be Beaten." *Countdown USA: Countdown to a Healthy Heart.* Allegheny General Hospital and Voluntary Hospitals of America, Inc., 1990.

"What Is Diabetes?" Canadian Diabetes Association (February 2, 1996). CDA Document ID: ADA037.

What Is Intensive Diabetes Management? Patient information. Diabetes Clinical Research Unit of Mount Sinai Hospital Toronto for Sherwood Medical Industries Canada Inc., distributed 1997.

"What You Should Know About Aspartame." International Food Information Council, 1100 Connecticut Avenue N.W., Suite 430, Washington D.C. 20036, November 4, 1996.

"What You Should Know About MSG." International Food Information Council, 1100 Connecticut Avenue N.W., Suite 430, Washington D.C. 20036, September 1991.

"What You Should Know About Sugars." International Food Information Council, 1100 Connecticut Avenue N.W., Suite 430, Washington D.C. 20036, May 1994.

"What's Your Type?" *News from the VIP*, No. 2 (Fall 1995): 1–2. Vitamin Information Program, Fine Chemicals Division of Hoffman-La Roche Ltd.

"When You Become an Amputee." Retrieved online from the Amputee Web Site (*www.amputee-online.ca*). July 2001.

Whitcomb, Randall. "The Key to Type 2." *Diabetes Dialogue*, Vol. 43, No. 4 (Winter 1996): 16–18.

Willett, W.C., et al. "Intake of Trans Fatty Acids and Risk of Coronary Heart Disease Among Women." *Lancet*, Vol. 341 (1993): 581–585.

Williamson, G.M., et al. "Social and Psychological Factors in Adjustment to Limb Amputation." *Journal of Social Behavior and Personality* 9 (1994): 249–268.

Williamson, Gail M. "Perceived Impact of Limb Amputation on Sexual Activity: A Study of Adult Amputees. "*The Journal of Sex Research*, Vol. 33, No. 3 (1996): 221–230.

Yale, Jean-Francois. "Glucose Results: Plasma or Whole Blood?" *Monitor*, Vol. 1 No. 2 (1997): 1-4.

"You Are What You Eat." *Equilibrium*, Issue 1 (1996): 16–20.

You Have Diabetes...Can You Have That? Booklet. Canadian Diabetes Association, distributed 1995.

Your Blood Sugar Level...What Does It Tell You? Patient information. Eli Lilly of Canada Inc., distributed 1997.

Your Diabetes Healthcare Team. *Equilibrium*, Issue 1 (1996): 34–36.

Your Kidneys. Patient information. The Kidney Foundation of Canada, distributed 1993.

Zinman, Bernard. "Insulin Analogues." *Diabetes Dialogue*, Vol. 43, No. 4 (Winter 1996): 14–15.

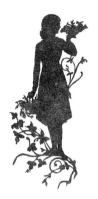

Index

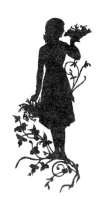

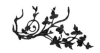

About the Author

M. Sara Rosenthal, Ph.D. is a bioethicist and sociologist with a long career as a medical health journalist. She received both her Masters and Ph.D. from The University of Toronto Joint Center for Bioethics, a World Health Organization Collaborating Center in bioethics. She is also an Associate of The University of Toronto Center for Health Promotion, also a WHO collaborating center in health promotion.

She is author of more than 25 widely recommended health books, including The Type 2 Diabetic Woman, 50 Ways to Manage *Type 2 Diabetes* and *The Canadian Type 2 Diabetes Sourcebook*. Her women's health titles include *The Gynecological Sourcebook*, recommended by *Ladies' Home Journal* and Women and Depression. Her work is translated into languages as diverse as Chinese and Arabic, and is reviewed and reprinted on more than 500 Websites, including WebMD. For more information, visit *www.sarahealth.com*.

Other Books by M. Sara Rosenthal

The Thyroid Sourcebook (4th edition, 2000)

The Gynecological Sourcebook (3rd edition, 1999)

The Pregnancy Sourcebook (3rd edition, 1999)

The Fertility Sourcebook (3rd edition, 2002)

The Breastfeeding Sourcebook (2nd edition, 1998)

The Breast Sourcebook (2nd edition, 1999)

The Gastrointestinal Sourcebook (1997; 1998)

The Type 2 Diabetic Woman (1999)

The Thyroid Sourcebook for Women (1999)

Women and Depression (2000)

Women of the '60s Turning 50 (Canada only; 2000)

Women and Passion (Canada only; 2000)

Managing PMS Naturally (2001)

Women Managing Stress (2002)

The Canadian Type 2 Diabetes Sourcebook
(Canada only; 2002)

The Hypothyroid Sourcebook (2002)

50 Ways Series

50 Ways To Prevent Colon Cancer (2000)

50 Ways Women Can Prevent Heart Disease (2000)

50 Ways To Manage Ulcer, Heartburn and Reflux (2001)

50 Ways To Manage Type 2 Diabetes (U.S. only; 2001)

50 Ways To Prevent and Manage Stress (2001)

50 Ways To Prevent Depression Without Drugs (2001)

SarahealthGuides™

These are M. Sara Rosenthal's own line of health books written by herself and other health authors. SarahealthGuides are dedicated to rare, controversial, or stigmatizing health topics you won't find in regular bookstores. SarahealthGuides are available only at online bookstores such as *amazon.com.* Visit *www.sarahealth.com* for upcoming titles.

Stopping Cancer At The Source (2001)

Women and Unwanted Hair (2001)

Living Well With Celiac Disease by Claudine Crangle (2002)

The Thyroid Cancer Book (2002)